I0473720

NIDDK
Prostate Research
Strategic Plan

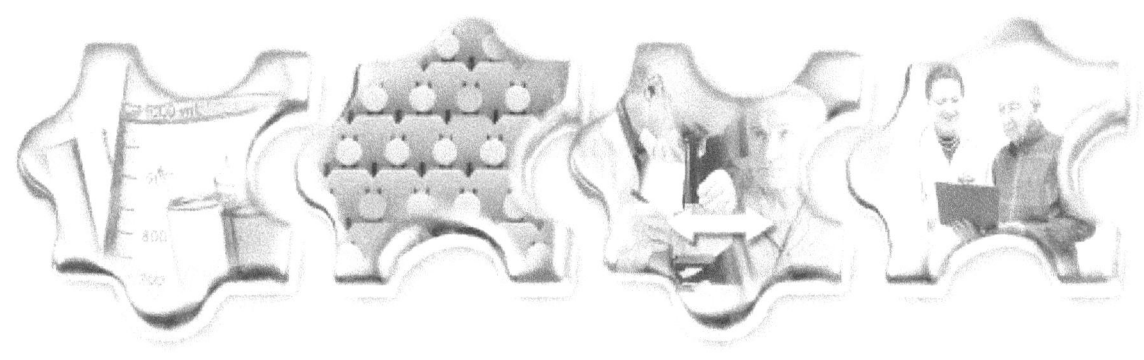

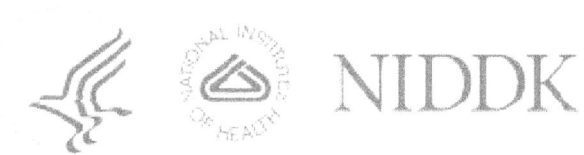

Department of Health and Human Services
National Institutes of Health
National Institute of Diabetes and Digestive and Kidney Diseases

Table of Contents

Foreword

The National Institute of Diabetes and Digestive and Kidney Diseases (NIDDK) is committed to supporting and promoting research in urologic disease as part of its mission to make important medical discoveries that improve health and save lives. Central to this is the Institute's focus on disorders of the prostate and the contribution of prostate biology to overall genito-urinary tract and pelvic floor physiology. The primary emphasis of the NIDDK's prostate research programs has traditionally been on benign disease. Principal among these are benign prostatic hyperplasia (BPH), along with the often associated lower urinary tract symptoms (LUTS), and prostatitis, especially chronic non-bacterial prostatitis (referred to as chronic prostatitis/chronic pelvic pain syndrome [CP/CPPS]). These disorders are common, chronic, and costly; they are found in all races and ethnic groups, and can affect men of all ages. In the case of BPH, symptoms increase in prevalence and severity as men age with nearly 50 percent of men experiencing LUTS by their sixth decade of life. In addition, benign prostate diseases result in significant morbidity and decreased quality of life and produce an enormous economic burden to patients and the nation from both direct health care costs and indirect costs, such as lost productivity.

Despite years of research, many fundamental questions remain unanswered regarding the underlying causes of benign prostate disorders and the factors associated with disease development and progression. For example, the relationship between histological and clinical BPH (i.e., symptomatic BPH) and the true contribution of prostate enlargement to LUTS are still debated. Also, there are no widely accepted strategies for preventing BPH/LUTS or objective criteria for early prognosis of disease progression to more severe outcomes, which often require surgical intervention. In the case of CP/CPPS, there is virtually no understanding of the etiology or pathophysiology of disease and there are no prevention strategies or generally effective therapies. Indeed, it even remains unclear as to the contribution of the prostate to the CP/CPPS hallmark symptom of chronic pelvic pain.

These long-standing, intractable questions concerning disease pathology and the need for increased progress in developing prevention and clinical care measures

prompted the NIDDK to examine the state-of-the-science and begin the process of developing a new vision to guide future research. To initiate this, the NIDDK convened an expert panel of clinical and basic scientists and epidemiologists in Chicago, Illinois, in the summer of 2006. This group reviewed the state of benign prostate research and the current priorities of the community and the NIDDK's prostate programs. Efforts were focused primarily on BPH/LUTS and CP/CPPS due to their relevance to the NIDDK mission. All those attending agreed that current funding and scientific trends suggested the field was in need of improved vitality and a renewed research focus. A number of the Chicago, Illinois participants became the nucleus of the NIDDK's Prostate Research Planning Committee.

In subsequent discussions from late 2006 through early 2007, the NIDDK Prostate Research Planning Committee, chaired by Dr. Steven Kaplan, outlined a process for developing a long-range agenda for benign prostate research. This included identification of a broad array of key scientific topics and areas of research to be evaluated for past progress and potential to advance our understanding of etiology, natural history/risk, and how best to prevent and treat benign prostate disorders. A diverse group of thought leaders representing basic scientists, epidemiologists, and clinical researchers were then identified and invited to participate in this effort. These individuals were charged with evaluating scientific topics/areas of research relevant to their specific expertise. This included identifying existing roadblocks to progress and opportunities for moving the field forward, as well as developing recommendations for new research efforts and for improving infrastructure and training.

In July 2007, the full group convened at the *NIDDK Prostate Basic and Clinical Science Strategic Planning Meeting* in Baltimore, Maryland, with a central goal of producing the basis of a document outlining a "strategic plan" for benign prostate disease research. It was agreed that this plan would identify questions of highest significance and provide consensus recommendations for addressing them, and by doing so would promote growth of the scientific community and enhance future research efforts. At this meeting, key scientific topics/areas of research were evaluated collectively and as part of four writing groups focused on basic research (co-chaired by Dr. Natasha Kyprianou and Dr. Wade Bushman); epidemiology of disease (co-chaired by Dr. Quentin Clemens and Dr. John Wei); translation of findings between the laboratory and the clinical setting (co-chaired by Dr. Robert Getzenberg and Dr. Scott Lucia); and clinical research (co-chaired by Dr. Claus G. Roehrborn, Dr. Steven Kaplan, and Dr. Kevin McVary). Concepts and recommendations originating at this meeting were then summarized and refined by the respective writing group co-chairs; the meeting chair, Dr. Kaplan; and the NIDDK over the next 6 months.

The present *NIDDK Prostate Research Strategic Plan* was developed directly through this collaborative effort and reflects the dedication and hard work of the many listed contributors. The strategic plan is organized into major sections representing four broad areas of research judged as critical for advancing the field: I. Basic Science; II. Epidemiology/Population-Based Studies; III. Translational Research; and IV. Clinical Sciences. These major sections are divided into chapters reflecting the scientific areas/topics of research discussed at the 2007 meeting in Baltimore, Maryland. This work serves as a guide for understanding past accomplishments and the current state of benign prostate research. More importantly, it provides research priorities and recommendations intended to focus and advance each scientific topic/area of research. In addition, each major section ends with a list of consensus high-priority recommendations. The Executive Summary serves as an overview of the plan's strategic vision and highlights key findings and recommendations. The *NIDDK Prostate Research Strategic Plan* is designed to be read by a broad audience of researchers, clinicians, advocacy groups, representatives from funding entities and, through our inclusion of lay/educational summaries, the patient community. The NIDDK will use recommendations and insights in this work to assist in developing future efforts addressing disease cause, prevention, and treatment. We hope it will also guide the research community and other health care professionals in addressing our common goal of improved care for patients suffering from benign disorders of the prostate.

The NIDDK wishes to thank all those who contributed to this Prostate Research Strategic Plan, as well as those who strive to understand and treat benign urologic disease.

Chris Mullins, Ph.D.
Director of Basic Cell Biology Programs in Urologic and
Kidney Disease
National Institute of Diabetes and Digestive and
Kidney Diseases
National Institutes of Health

Planning Committee

Steven Kaplan, M.D., Planning Committee Chair
Weill Medical College of Cornell University

Wade Bushman, M.D., Ph.D.
University of Wisconsin-Madison

J. Quentin Clemens, M.D.
University of Michigan

Michael Freeman, Ph.D.
Children's Hospital, Boston, Harvard Medical School

Robert Getzenberg, Ph.D.
The Johns Hopkins University

Natasha Kyprianou, Ph.D.
University of Kentucky

M. Scott Lucia, M.D.
University of Colorado

Kevin McVary, M.D.
Northwestern University

Claus G. Roehrborn, M.D.
University of Texas Southwestern

John Wei, M.D.
University of Michigan

NIDDK Program Staff

Chris Mullins, Ph.D.
DKUH, NIDDK, NIH

Leroy M. Nyberg, Jr., M.D., Ph.D.
DKUH, NIDDK, NIH

NIDDK Technical Writer and Editor

Ms. Emily Tinkler
DKUH, NIDDK, NIH

List of Contributors

Michael Barry, M.D.
Chief
General Medicine Unit
Massachusetts General Hospital
Boston, MA

Wade Bushman, M.D., Ph.D.
Robert F. and Dolores K. Schnoes Chair
Urologic Research
Department of Surgery
Division of Urology
University of Wisconsin Hospital and Clinics
Madison, WI

J. Quentin Clemens, M.D.
Associate Professor
Department of Urology
University of Michigan Medical Center
Ann Arbor, MI

Mark Day, Ph.D.
Professor
Department of Urology
University of Michigan
Ann Arbor, MI

Renty Franklin, Ph.D.
Professor
Biomedical Sciences/Dental School
University of Maryland Baltimore
Baltimore, MD

Michael Freeman, Ph.D.
Director
Urologic Research
Department of Urology
Children's Hospital Boston
Boston, MA

Robert H. Getzenberg, Ph.D.
Research Director
James Buchanan Brady Urological Institute
Professor of Urology
The Johns Hopkins University School of
    Medicine
Baltimore, MD

Simon Hayward, Ph.D.
Associate Professor
Department of Urologic Surgery
Vanderbilt University Medical Center
Nashville, TN

Steven Jacobsen, M.D., Ph.D.
Director of Research
Department of Research and Evaluation
Kaiser Permanente Southern California
Pasadena, CA

David Jarrard, M.D.
Department of Surgery
Division of Urology
University of Wisconsin
Madison, WI

Steven Kaplan, M.D.
Professor of Urology
Weill Medical College of Cornell University
New York, NY

Tracey Krupski, M.D., M.P.H.
Assistant Professor of Urology
Department of Surgery
Division of Urology
Duke University
Raleigh, NC

John Kusek, Ph.D.
Director
Renal and Urology Clinical Trials
Division of Kidney, Urologic, and Hematologic
    Diseases
National Institute of Diabetes and Digestive and
    Kidney Diseases
National Institutes of Health
Bethesda, MD

Natasha Kyprianou, Ph.D.
Professor
Department of Surgery
Division of Urology
University of Kentucky
Lexington, KY

John Lavelle, M.B., F.R.C.S.I.
Associate Professor
Department of Surgery
Division of Urology
University of North Carolina at Chapel Hill
Chapel Hill, NC

Jeannette Lee, Ph.D.
Professor of Medicine, Hematology, and Oncology
University of Alabama at Birmingham
Birmingham, AL

Franklin Lowe, M.D., M.P.H.
Professor of Clinical Urology
Department of Urology
St. Luke's/Roosevelt Hospital
Columbia University
New York, NY

M. Scott Lucia, M.D.
Director
Prostate Diagnostic Laboratory
Associate Professor of Pathology
Department of Pathology
University of Colorado Health Sciences Center
Aurora, CO

Jill Macoska, Ph.D.
Associate Professor and Associate Chair for
    Translational Research
Department of Urology
University of Michigan
Ann Arbor, MI

4

Robert Matusik, Ph.D.
Professor and Director
Vanderbilt Prostate Cancer Center
Department of Urologic Surgery
Vanderbilt University Medical Center
Nashville, TN

Kevin McKenna, Ph.D.
Professor
Departments of Physiology and Urology
Feinberg School of Medicine
Northwestern University
Chicago, IL

Kevin McVary, M.D., F.A.C.S.
Professor
Department of Urology
Feinberg School of Medicine
Northwestern University
Chicago, IL

Chris Mullins, Ph.D.
Director
Basic Cell Biology Programs in Urologic and Kidney
    Disease
Division of Kidney, Urologic, and Hematologic
    Diseases
National Institute of Diabetes and Digestive
    and Kidney Diseases
National Insititutes of Health
Bethesda, MD

Peter Nelson, M.D.
Associate Professor
Department of Medicine and Oncology
Fred Hutchinson Cancer Research Center
Seattle, WA

J. Curtis Nickel, M.D.
Professor of Urology
Department of Urology
Queen's University
Kingston General Hospital
Kingston, Ontario, Canada

Leroy M. Nyberg, Jr., M.D., Ph.D.
Director
Urology Programs
Division of Kidney, Urologic, and Hematologic
    Diseases
National Institute of Diabetes and Digestive and
    Kidney Diseases
National Institutes of Health
Bethesda, MD

J. Kellogg Parsons, M.D., M.H.S.
Assistant Professor
Department of Surgery
Division of Urology
University of California, San Diego
San Diego, CA

Donna Peehl, Ph.D.
Associate Professor
Department of Urology
Stanford University
Stanford Medical Center
Stanford, CA

Michel Pontari, M.D.
Professor of Urology
Department of Urology
Temple University School of Medicine
Philadelphia, PA

Claus G. Roehrborn, M.D.
Professor and Chair
Department of Urology
University of Texas Southwestern Medical Center
    at Dallas
Dallas, TX

David Rowley, Ph.D.
Professor
Department of Molecular and Cellular Biology
Baylor College of Medicine
Houston, TX

Aruna Sarma, Ph.D.
Research Assistant Professor
Department of Urology
University of Michigan
Ann Arbor, MI

Robert A. Star, M.D.
Director
Division of Kidney, Urologic, and Hematologic
    Diseases
National Institute of Diabetes and Digestive and
    Kidney Diseases
National Institutes of Health
Bethesda, MD

Alexis Te, M.D.
Associate Professor of Urology
Director
Brady Prostate Center
Department of Urology
Weill Medical College of Cornell
    University
New York, NY

Emily Tinkler
Technical Writer and Editor
Division of Kidney, Urologic, and Hematologic
    Diseases
National Institute of Diabetes and Digestive and
    Kidney Diseases
National Institutes of Health
Bethesda, MD

Kathleen C. Torkko, Ph.D.
Instructor
Department of Pathology
University of Colorado Denver School of Medicine
Aurora, CO

Zhou Wang, Ph.D.
Director
Urological Research
Professor
Department of Urology
Shadyside Medical Center
University of Pittsburgh
Pittsburgh, PA

John Wei, M.D., M.S.
Associate Professor of Urology
Department of Urology
University of Michigan
Ann Arbor, MI

Lynette Wilson, Ph.D.
Associate Professor
Department of Cell Biology
New York University School of Medicine
New York, NY

6

enign diseases of the prostate are among the most common urologic diseases seen by health care professionals. Two of the most significant prostate disorders, based on a variety of troubling symptoms and resulting in diminished quality of life (QOL) of affected males are benign prostate hyperplasia (BPH) and prostatitis (see Table below for descriptions of common benign prostate diseases covered in this document). BPH, which is often associated with a collection of lower urinary tract symptoms (LUTS), affects men of all races and ethnic groups and can progress in severity over time. If untreated, BPH can lead to significant consequences, such as acute urinary retention, incontinence, and urinary tract infection. Pathologically, 50 percent of men in their 50s will have prostatic hyperplasia and 26 to 46 percent of men will have moderate to severe LUTS between the ages of 40 to 79 years. In 2000, more than 4.4 million office and outpatient hospital visits involved a primary diagnosis of BPH and another 3.4 million visits included BPH as a secondary diagnosis. In that same year, the total direct cost (meaning costs associated with direct care, such as office visits) of BPH was estimated to be $1.1 billion, while expenditure on outpatient prescription drugs is approximately $194 million annually. The total cost to society, including indirect costs (meaning costs resulting from disease, such as lost productivity) in the United States, has been estimated to be as high as $4 billion annually. Prostatitis affects men of all ages and leads to significant bother and diminished QOL. Prostatitis comprises four categories of acute or chronic disease, including chronic prostatitis/chronic pelvic pain syndrome (CP/CPPS). Despite its relatively high prevalence (estimates have ranged from 2.7 to 9.7 percent in men 18 years and older), prostatitis remains a poorly understood disorder and is very challenging to treat. Moreover, prostatitis, specifically in its chronic form CP/CPPS, can be physically and psychologically devastating for many patients. For example, the QOL for a patient with chronic prostatitis has been reported to be similar to that experienced by patients with certain forms of heart disease or active Crohn's disease.

Common Benign Prostate Disorders: Classifications and Symptom Profiles*
Benign Prostatic Hyperplasia (BPH)
Commonly characterized by prostate enlargement due to nonmalignant proliferation of glandular (e.g., epithelial) and stromal (e.g., smooth muscle) cells (to varying degrees). BPH can be further subgrouped as histological BPH and clinical BPH: <ul><li>**Histological BPH** is defined by the presence of an increased number of epithelial and stromal cells in the periurethral area of the prostate upon histological examination. Histological BPH may or may not be associated with symptoms.</li><li>**Clinical BPH** (also referred to as symptomatic BPH) is defined by the presence of some or all of a diverse array of lower urinary tract symptoms (LUTS). LUTS includes (but is not limited to) storage problems such as frequency, nocturia, urgency, and urge incontinence or emptying problems such as hesitancy, poor stream, and post-void dribbling. These symptoms have traditionally been thought to be a result of obstruction of the prostatic urethra, though clinical BPH may or may not involve a significant enlargement of the prostate.</li></ul>
Prostatitis
Commonly characterized in general terms as inflammation of the prostate gland. However, prostatitis is more often discussed in relation to the following classification scheme: <ul><li>**Category I.** **Acute bacterial prostatitis.** This acute form of prostatitis is associated with the presence of a uropathogen and symptoms of bacterial infection.</li><li>**Category II.** **Chronic bacterial prostatitis.** This chronic form of prostatitis involves a chronic bacterial infection of the prostate with or without symptoms of infection.</li><li>**Category III.** **Chronic prostatitis/chronic pelvic pain syndrome (CP/CPPS).** CP/CPPS is characterized by chronic pain in the pelvic area, lacks a detectable uropathogen, and is sometimes associated with urinary symptoms and sexual dysfunction. The disease etiology and the source of the pain (i.e., the prostate or other pelvic tissue) are not known for CP/CPPS.</li><li>**Category IV.** **Asymptomatic inflammatory prostatitis.** This form of prostatitis is characterized by evidence of prostate inflammation but absence of symptoms.</li></ul>
* These descriptions are not meant as updates of published disease definitions, but are general characterizations for reference in this specific work.

Health care professionals have access to findings from a variety of basic, epidemiological, and clinical research study results, and a wide spectrum of treatments shown to be effective for some patients (e.g., current medical therapies for BPH/LUTS). Yet, there is a lack of information to effectively progress from the realm of diagnosis and treatment into the realm of prevention (or earlier treatment). For example, it would be enormously useful if clinicians could identify men in early adulthood who are at risk for developing BPH/LUTS and then alter the natural history of the disease process through preventative therapy. In addition, some benign prostate conditions such as CP/CPPS are especially poorly understood at all levels, including the fundamental causes (i.e., etiology) and the natural history of disease. Such deficiencies have slowed the development of generally effective treatment options for CP/CPPS.

As the population ages and the health burden for prostate-related disorders increases, there is a need to develop a long-range strategic plan to focus and direct efforts to better understand benign prostate diseases. Efforts to provide improved research and clinical observations will be of major benefit to investigators, health care professionals, institutional providers of care, and those suffering from prostate-related disorders. In recognition of these significant challenges, the National Institute of Diabetes and Digestive and Kidney Diseases (NIDDK) convened an expert panel of key opinion leaders that included a broad spectrum of basic researchers, translational scientists, epidemiologists, and clinicians and clinical researchers, to formulate a strategic plan for research in benign prostate disease. The overall statement of purpose of this collaborative effort is "to discuss, evaluate, and propose research needs and a long-range research agenda (a "strategic plan") for NIDDK grant portfolios related to research into benign prostate disease." The underlying principle of this effort is to *focus on quality and direction of the science.* Eventual implementation of this strategic plan will require a partnership of stakeholders, including the scientific community, the Federal Government, and other public and private organizations and institutions.

This focused group of research and thought leaders identified four major areas of key significance for future investigation: 1) Basic Science (i.e., the study of fundamental biological aspects of a process or disease); 2) Epidemiology/Population-Based Studies (i.e., the study of factors affecting the health of a population);

3) Translational Opportunities (i.e., the movement of findings and insights between the laboratory and clinical care); and 4) Clinical Sciences (i.e., the assessment of disease features and development of treatments). There is great opportunity within these four areas to compare and translate findings for benign prostate diseases and related syndromes between the research laboratory and the clinical setting. This implies and requires new ideas and directions for moving insights from the laboratory to clinical trials or practice and back. In addition, current roadblocks must be identified and overcome. For example, at-risk populations must be better defined and novel technologies need to be applied to these disease settings. Currently, there are too few well-characterized resources or specimen banks available with which to move studies between the bench and the bedside. Furthermore, there are too few established investigators and multidisciplinary teams to address these issues.

The following *NIDDK Prostate Research Strategic Plan* represents a blueprint that investigators and the Federal Government can use to identify where the field has been, where the field is now and, most importantly, where future research efforts should be directed. Not surprisingly, there is overlap in the major sections comprising this document with respect to some topics and recommendations. This overlap does not imply redundancy; rather it reflects how these four areas of research are synergistic and highly interdependent. The challenge will be to create a more dynamic stream of communication between these areas to improve integration of research findings and advance patient care through research.

The strategic plan is by no means all encompassing or definitive. Research is always fluid, and this document should be viewed as a work in progress. Ultimately, change can only come from those determined and destined to undertake it. As Albert Einstein noted, "The process of scientific discovery is, in effect, a continual flight from wonder." Those who have contributed to this work hope that it will serve as a blueprint for scientific discovery in benign prostate disease in the future.

The overall goals and missions, along with key scientific recommendations and priorities, of the four major areas of focus of the strategic plan are summarized briefly on the following pages.

I. BASIC SCIENCE

Overall Goal and Mission

Basic science research efforts are predicated on integrating clinical and translational approaches to benign prostate disease. Specific areas that are undergoing the most rapid change, as well as receiving increasing recognition for their importance, involve studies of pain, inflammation, and neural and vascular biology. To ensure productive integration of basic science research with translational efforts, a corresponding evolution in the focus of basic science research must occur. In addition, there is a critical need for basic science investigators to generate insights that can inform clinical research and drive the development of new paradigms that will refine categorization, study, and eventually, a fundamental understanding of poorly described clinical entities such as BPH and prostatitis. Thus, in the context of benign prostate disease one can define the potential contributions of basic research to the clinical setting principally in two arenas: 1) development of appropriate disease-relevant pathways, proteins, and biochemical events, opening the way for application of "smart" (i.e., targeted) therapies based on known physiological insights; and 2) identification of biomarkers that improve diagnosis, categorization, and prognosis of disease.

Research Priorities and Recommendations

Development

- Elucidate the mechanisms that provide for integrated regulation of cell proliferation, differentiation, and homeostasis.

Vascular Biology

- Determine mechanisms that control prostate vascularity.

Metabolism

- Apply metabolomics approaches to studies of both normal and diseased prostate tissues.
- Assess the changes in intermediary metabolism, bioenergetics, and proliferation that may contribute to the development of disease.

Inflammation and Reactive Stroma

- Understand the etiology of prostatic inflammation.
- Describe how inflammation contributes to the proliferative/hyperplastic or prostatitis-type phenotypes.
- Observe molecular interactions between the various types of immune cells in the human prostate (e.g., granulocytes, lymphocytes, monocytes, and macrophages) and prostate epithelial, stromal fibroblast, and endothelial cells.

Stem Cells

- Identify and characterize stem and progenitor cells for the stromal and epithelial compartments of the prostate.
- Determine the lineages and hierarchies in stromal and epithelial compartments and the interactions between them that regulate the process of growth and differentiation.

Hormonal Effects

- Elucidate the hormonal effects on specific epithelial and stromal progenitor cells and lineages.
- Understand the aging effect on androgen- and/or estrogen-responsive genes in the prostate.

Animal Models

- Develop new rodent models to test therapeutic treatment during the disease processes, as well as methods to relieve symptoms after the urologic disorder is established.

Aging

- Elucidate the link between aging, BPH, prostatitis, and prostate cancer.

Signaling

- Characterize disease-relevant pathways, proteins, and biochemical events, opening the way for application of "smart" (i.e., targeted) therapy based on known physiological mechanisms.
- Identify disease biomarkers that allow proper diagnosis, disease categorization, and clinically relevant prognostic information.

Neurobiology

- Understand the role of adrenergic activity in benign prostate growth.
- Identify the mechanisms by which innervation regulates benign growth.

Proteomics and New Technologies

- Establish approaches and standards for the comprehensive (or at a minimum, high-throughput) measurement of multiple proteins/protein modifications.

Infrastructure Needs

- *Human Tissue*
  Collect and bank human tissues from patients of various ages for the study of benign prostate diseases, as well as other urologic diseases. Continue development of centralized tissue resources with open access.
- *Interdisciplinary Research*
  Promote interdisciplinary research that focuses on the mechanisms linking benign prostate diseases that occur in parallel with other organ-specific diseases and systemic conditions, including metabolic syndrome, cardiovascular disease, diabetes, and erectile dysfunction.

- *Training and Fellowship Programs*
Establish training programs that encourage young investigators to pursue careers in benign prostate research. These efforts would be aided by increasing the visibility and recognition of this research—something that might be most effectively communicated by promoting interdisciplinary research and developing a high-profile scientific venue. There should be a special effort to bring together independent basic scientists and clinical fellows and junior faculty to develop collaborative and bidirectional research efforts. Increase fellowship funding opportunities for urologists to pursue basic science training and create mechanisms that require collaborations between urologists, other clinicians, and basic scientists. This recommendation is key to achieving specific milestones for progress in the field.
- *New Meeting Venue*
There is a need to elevate the visibility of prostate biology and lower urinary tract disease research. One recommendation is to establish a Gordon Conference focused on prostate biology and benign lower urinary tract disease.

High-Priority Recommendations

Clinically defined BPH and prostatitis often involve changes in bladder function, pelvic floor function, and neural function, and may co-exist with other systemic conditions. These associated conditions may be as important as the changes occurring in the prostate. These insights call for the development of new clinical paradigms and comprehensive research approaches. The targeted priorities are the following:
- Create new models for the study of benign disease.
- Develop a comprehensive understanding of the signaling, interaction, and cross talk between multiple cell types in the prostate.
- Understand the effect of aging on prostate biology and lower urogenital system function.
- Apply new technologies and imaging techniques.
- Diversify efforts to establish points of biological congruence between cell and animal models and the human prostate that will facilitate translational research.
- Characterize disease-relevant cellular pathways to open the way for application of "smart" (i.e., targeted) therapies based on known physiological mechanisms.
- Encourage an integrated and multifaceted study of endocrine regulation of lower urogenital biology.

- Promote training and career development efforts for investigators interested in research careers in benign prostate disease.

II. EPIDEMIOLOGY/ POPULATION-BASED STUDIES

Overall Goal and Mission

The primary goal of this field is to apply epidemiology and population-based sciences and health services research in multidisciplinary teams to the study of the etiology, management, and outcomes of benign prostate disease. A key impediment to progress in this field is the lack of specificity of current diagnoses and definitions of benign prostate diseases, which focus on symptoms rather than underlying etiology. Although observational studies generate insights into the burden and etiologic mechanisms of benign prostatic disease, further evaluation of these mechanisms are then required in the laboratory or in a clinical trial setting. Conversely, observations made in the laboratory or in a clinical trial require implementation strategies to properly document the dissemination and cost-effective use of novel interventions into practice. To circumvent these hurdles, population scientists will have to partner with basic and clinical scientists to change the existing paradigm and develop disease classifications based on knowledge of etiology.

Research Priorities and Recommendations

Epidemiology of Prostatitis
- Assess the natural history of disease.
- Promote studies of minority groups.

Epidemiology of Benign Prostatic Hyperplasia
- Encourage longitudinal studies of the natural history of BPH.
- Improve disease classifications based on underlying etiology, including hormonal levels and balance; assessment of neurologic and bladder functions; and genetic testing for predisposition and determinations of protein expression.
- Identify risk factors, particularly modifiable risk factors that may serve as potential targets for clinical intervention.

Practice Patterns for Benign Prostatic Hyperplasia and Prostatitis
- Identify reproducible and widely accepted quality of care indicators.
- Promote efforts and studies to establish guidelines acceptable to both urologists and primary care physicians.

- Encourage urologic researchers interested in examining clinical epidemiology, economics, and quality of care.

- Address differences in benign prostate disease management guidelines between different organizations and between the United States and Europe.

- Understand variables that include provider characteristics, patient characteristics, marketing, the media, the Internet, and sociologic pressures to potentially optimize the efficient delivery of the latest, most effective, and most cost-efficient health care for BPH and CP/CPPS.

- Develop user-friendly QOL instruments and condition-specific measures of lower urinary tract dysfunctions.

- Provide prospective assessment of the direct and indirect costs and cost effectiveness of contemporary treatment modalities for BPH and CP/CPPS over the long term. This can be done using administrative datasets or larger population-based cohort studies.
- Develop strategies to disseminate cost-effectiveness data and teach clinicians to use therapies in a more cost-efficient manner.

- Correlate treatment response to known past medical risk factors in men with either BPH or prostatitis. This also should include implementing evidence-based medicine into decision making and ascertaining the influence of costs/reimbursements on management decisions related to BPH and CP/CPPS.

High Priority Recommendations

- Develop classification schemes for benign prostate disease based on new insights into underlying etiology.
- Develop data and tissue resources that contain well-characterized population-based information necessary for investigation of risk factors, natural history, etiologic mechanisms, QOL, quality of care, and decision making for benign prostate disease.
- Communicate the importance of rigorous clinical research methodologies when applied in the basic, clinical, and population-based settings.
- Ensure that high-quality study designs are used to generate and test hypotheses of key significance to benign prostatic disease.
- Disseminate clinical trial findings, medical and surgical therapies, evidence-based medicine, and use of health-related QOL measures into clinical practice.
- Train and mentor epidemiologists, health services researchers, clinical investigators, and students interested in the study of benign prostate disease.

III. TRANSLATIONAL OPPORTUNITIES

Overall Goal and Mission

The primary goal of research focused on benign prostatic diseases is to advance the clinical care of patients suffering from these disorders. Translational research involves the bidirectional movement of scientific insights and concepts between the basic research laboratory and the clinical setting. The mission of the translational opportunities group is to integrate basic science, epidemiological/population-based studies, and clinical science to promote important directions and common resources for translational research. Key areas of interest are the development of novel biomarkers and therapeutic approaches for these diseases.

Research Priorities and Recommendations

Overall Infrastructure Needs

- Establish functional basic scientist-clinician research relationships. Institutional incentives and research opportunities need to be ongoing, formalized, and encouraged by the academic community and its partners.

Serum and Tissue Biorepositories for Prostatic Disease

- Continue efforts to establish tissue, serum, and urine biorepositories from large multi-center clinical trials. These would create unique and opportune resources for translational research. Also, the collection and archiving of sera, urine, and/or tissue during patient management and clinical trials should be promoted.

- Develop new and ongoing database resources for benign prostate disease. Opportunities include the further description, characterization, and advertising of databases for prostatic disease that currently exist (e.g., bioinformatics networks). Additional opportunities include the further examination of current databases to help identify risk factors, prognostic variables, and longitudinal changes in function and QOL for both treated and natural history patients.

- Determine whether histologic changes (e.g., inflammatory, composition, and angiogenesis) correlate with disease severity and risk of progression in BPH/LUTS, as well as the potential role for prostate biopsy and immunohistochemistry in the evaluation of progression, risk, and treatment response in BPH/LUTS.

- Develop serum, semen, and/or urine-based biomarkers; genomic and/or proteomic signatures; and tissue-based markers to help identify men at risk of developing symptoms of BPH and CP/CPPS and men at risk for progressive disease.
- Develop imaging approaches to assess disease severity and risk of progression based upon biomarker results.

- Create studies using normal tissue for BPH as the benign comparator to prostate cancer. Also, standardized, nonsubjective disease definitions must be developed to allow genetic studies to be productive.
- Examine epigenetic changes in men with BPH or CP/CPPS for the purpose of establishing expression patterns and potential biomarkers and therapeutic targets.

High-Priority Recommendations

- Develop standardized clinically significant benign prostate disease/syndrome definitions that may be characterized by measurable phenotypic features.
- Define commonalities (e.g., pathological, clinical, and molecular) that are shared between clinical syndromes (e.g., BPH, pelvic pain, prostatitis, etc.).
- Encourage standardized institutional archiving by:
  - Using uniform protocols and database fields.
  - Networking and/or pooling with other institutions.
  - Creating common platform pools (serum/tissue arrays).

- Determine whether treatments that target inflammation, angiogenesis, or both inhibit the development of BPH nodules and alter the pathology on biopsy (using histopathology or immunohistochemistry measurements).
- Investigate the relationship between histological changes with disease severity and risk for progression for BPH/LUTS.
- Develop and identify serum, semen, and/or urine-based biomarkers, as well as genomic/proteomic signatures that can identify progressive BPH, identify men at risk of developing symptomatic BPH, distinguish various etiologic mechanisms of prostatitis, and be used to identify novel therapeutic targets.

IV. CLINICAL SCIENCES

Overall Goal and Mission

The clinical study of benign prostate disease represents an important and dynamic area of research. There are many research questions for these very common conditions that remain largely unanswered. The clinical sciences section intends to develop a prioritized list of recommendations and priorities for clinical research related to benign disorders associated with the prostate (e.g., BPH, prostatitis, and CP/CPPS), the broadly defined LUTS, and general male pelvic health-related diseases. This section also makes recommendations for improving the infrastructure needed to facilitate clinical research, including the infrastructure required to conduct and monitor clinical trials.

Research opportunities in the clinical study of benign prostate disease should be addressed in multiple tiers. Key questions need to be the focus of these studies. For example, what is the typical phenotype of patients who present with benign prostate disease? This assessment includes age, type of LUTS, prostate size, presence of inflammation, type of tissue within the prostate (e.g., glands, muscular, or fibrous tissues, etc.), as well as existing co-morbid conditions like diabetes and obesity. Also, are there more effective ways that health care workers can easily identify patients at risk or likely to have progression of disease? Research into reliable biomarkers and imaging techniques are fertile areas of investigation to address these questions.

One current area of weakness in our ability to accurately diagnose and assess the severity of benign prostate disease is the lack of reliable and consistent outcome measurements. This will require a multidisciplinary effort designed to better define disease states and therapeutic benefits. This also will require more consistent and reproducible clinical trial designs to assess disease prevention, progression of disease, and responses to therapy. The use of clinical trial registration and wide dissemination of trial protocols will be very helpful towards achieving these goals. Therapeutic areas to be examined should include behavioral and lifestyle alteration, including diet and exercise, phototherapy, plant extracts, medical therapies either alone or in combination, and minimally invasive surgical therapies.

Research Priorities and Recommendations

Defining the Clinical Phenotypes for Benign Prostate Disease

Consider important issues in evaluating the disease phenotype of patients with benign prostate disorders. Such issues include:

* Age
* Urinating symptom type (i.e., storage versus voiding)
* Prostate size
* Presence of inflammation
* Histology and cellular pathology
* Imaging findings
* Co-morbid conditions

Promote studies assessing disease phenotypes based on the following:

* Pain
* Presence of urinary symptoms

Association of Benign Prostate Disease with Co-morbid Conditions

Evaluate disease relationships of the following conditions:

* LUTS and sexual dysfunction
* Metabolic syndrome, LUTS, and sexual dysfunction
* Metabolic syndrome, low testosterone, and pelvic health

Measuring Disease Severity and Outcomes

* Develop instruments to assess lower urinary tract dysfunction related to males (or perhaps both males and females) including the impact on health status and QOL.

Clinical Trial Design

* Establish new disease-specific registries and collaborative networks (including web-based resources).
* Assess combination therapy in the treatment of prostate disorders.
* Promote the study of primary prevention for benign prostate diseases.

* Develop specific clinical trial concepts, including medical therapy, phytotherapy, behavioral and lifestyle interventions, and minimally invasive surgical therapies.

High-Priority Recommendations

* Make obesity and lifestyle interventions a priority area for benign prostate disease.
    - Study specific hypotheses of how BPH/LUTS is impacted by obesity, the metabolic syndrome, and related diseases.
    - Organize and promote collaborative efforts between urologists, clinical trial experts, exercise physiologists, and dietary experts.
    - Assess the relationship between the various manifestations of metabolic syndrome and BPH/LUTS.
* Develop preventive strategies aimed at underlying common pathophysiology of benign prostate disease.
* Develop studies that assess disease "phenotypes" and lead to better disease definitions (e.g., size versus morphological characteristics and their relative importance in producing symptoms, obstructive versus irritative symptoms relative to prostate morphology and size, and CP/CPPS patient phenotypes relative to urologic symptom profiles).
* Encourage the study of primary prevention for CP/CPPS and BPH/LUTS.
* Develop a plan for a multidisciplinary working group to develop a specific research agenda for symptom and health status measurement related to male LUTS.
    - Include investigators interested in the broad spectrum of underlying conditions, as well as the developers of the prominent instruments.
    - Invite professional societies, national and international, and other Government organizations to participate.
* Develop a collaborative network to standardize treatment assessment.
    - Create a LUTS Treatment Collaborative Network that would allow the critical aggregation of thought leaders, trial design experts, industrial collaborators, and various Federal agencies to identify clinically meaningful assessments of promising medical, minimally invasive, and surgical treatments.

Steven Kaplan, M.D.
Planning Committee Chair
Weill Medical College of Cornell University

I. Basic Science

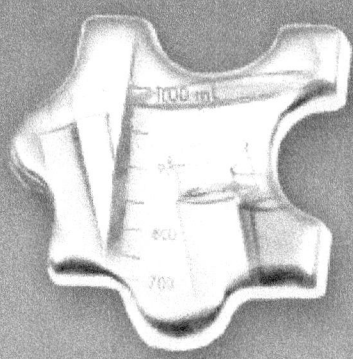

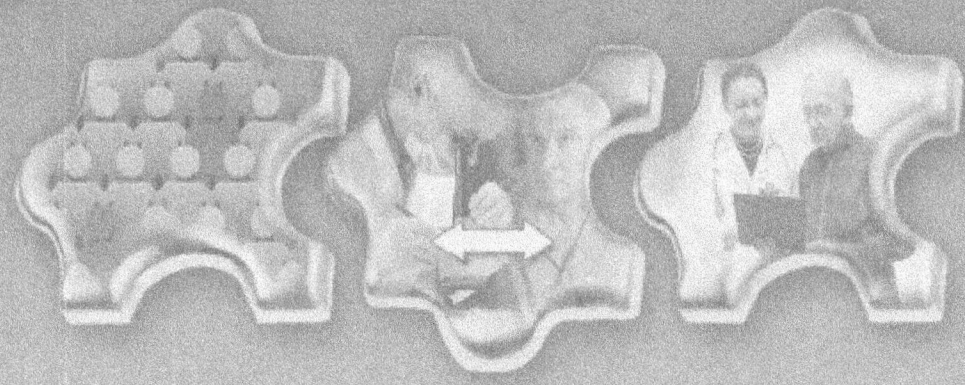

Mission Statement

The clinical and translational approaches to studying benign prostate disease are undergoing a rapid evolution with increasing importance being attached to studies of pain, inflammation, neural, and vascular considerations. To ensure productive integration of basic science with translational efforts, a corresponding evolution in the focus of basic science research must occur. The topics discussed within this section include recommendations for further work along established lines of inquiry, but also stress the need for novel approaches and new areas of investigation. In addition, there is a critical need for basic science investigators to generate insights that can inform clinical research and drive the development of new paradigms that will refine categorization, study, and understanding of poorly circumscribed clinical entities such as benign prostatic hyperplasia (BPH) and prostatitis. A key feature of these efforts is to examine the important relationships with adjacent organs and to recognize that prostate disease may involve systemic conditions or shared disease processes affecting multiple organs.

800

700

600

asic research may be described as research that examines the fundamental aspects of biology or, in the case of disease-oriented research, the underlying causes of disease. To understand how basic science relates to benign prostate disease, it is helpful to include a background that provides the definitions and the purpose of basic science, including what this area of research seeks to discover and improve. Benign prostate disease represents a group of common disorders involving diverse symptoms. These disorders affect men of all ages, but many are associated with the aging process. Based on the particular disorder, symptoms may include pain and/ or any of a variety of lower urinary tract symptoms (LUTS), such as difficulty urinating. These symptoms, often attributed to enlargement or inflammation of the prostate, are extremely common. However, the fundamental cause(s) of these symptoms remains largely unknown. Previous research efforts have provided key insights into the mechanisms that may contribute to prostate enlargement. In addition, clinical studies have shown that aging; changes in the nervous, immunological, and/or the circulatory systems; and defects in metabolism may play equally important roles.

Based on knowledge learned from past research efforts, this section describes a vision for the future of basic research relevant to understanding the origin of benign prostate growth and disease, as well as LUTS and other relevant symptoms. Combining scientific approaches is considered a key feature of future basic research. This strategy will help to address the complex nature of the benign prostate conditions and serve as the basis for the development of more effective therapeutic interventions and new predictors of disease. The potential contributions of basic research to the clinical setting in the context of benign prostate disease lie principally in two arenas: 1) understanding disease-relevant pathways, proteins, and biochemical events, opening the way for application of more appropriate and effective therapies based on known physiological insights; and 2) identifying disease biomarkers that allow proper diagnosis, disease categorization, and clinically relevant predictive information.

The goal of this basic science section is to identify facets of basic prostate research that are priorities for future work and to attempt to relate those to the clinical features of benign prostatic disease. Recent molecular technology advances enable basic scientists to explore beyond the boundaries of current understanding as it relates to clinical urologic conditions. Novel bioinformatics tools and databases, knowledge of functional roles of proteins and protein modifications, new imaging tools that allow high resolution of cellular and tissue events, and mass spectrometric techniques will permit extensive and precise analysis of cellular molecules on a large scale. In the table shown, the left column contains a list of the clinical features of benign prostatic disease, and the right column contains a list of key facets of basic biology research.

Research Focus

- Prostate growth
- Bladder response to obstruction
- Pelvic floor response to obstruction
- Symptoms:
  – Frequency
  – Pain
  – Sexual function
- Metabolism
- Inflammation/Microbiology
- Sensation
- Hormonal influences
- Drug action

- Prostate stem cells
- Cell-cell interactions
- Embryology
- Animal and cell models
- Vasculature
- Hormonal action
- Signaling cascades
- Inflammation
- Aging
- Metabolism
- Neuronal influences
- Genetics and genomics
- Proteomics
- New technologies

Three major themes are reflected in the following individual chapters:

I. An integrative approach to the study of prostate growth regulation. The key areas of study are:

- Prostate stem cells
- Cell-cell interactions and tissue microenvironment
- Embryology
- Vasculature
- Intermediary metabolism
- Hormonal action
- Signaling cascades
- Animal and cell models

II. An integrative approach to the study of inflammation and aging. The key areas of study are:

- Prostate stem cells and senescence
- Epigenetics
- Microenvironment
- Vascular biology

- Metabolism
- Hormonal action
- Signaling cascades
- Animal models

III. Efforts to identify and investigate causes of lower urogenital tract dysfunction. The key areas of study are:

- Inflammation
- Aging
- Metabolism
- Neuronal influences

A highlighted recommended avenue for future work is to engage in multidisciplinary approaches to examine processes such as inflammation or aging in disease and especially symptom-driven diseases. A second highlighted recommendation is to use basic science insights to enable or even drive paradigm-shifts in studies of the etiology, manifestation, and natural history of benign prostate diseases.

1. Development

The study of prostate development has provided many important insights into prostate growth regulation. Key areas of established knowledge include the role of androgen signaling and estrogen signaling in normal prostate development; identification of many important signaling pathways and transcription factors that control morphogenesis, cell proliferation, and differentiation; and the role of stem cells, progenitor cells, and basal cells.[1,2] The stage of development, with solid undifferentiated epithelial cords in the distal region and a forming lumen and cellular differentiation in the proximal region, reflects the early postnatal period in rodent prostate development (Figure 1).

Studies of prostate development should provide the basis to examine the role of developmental regulators in the aging and inflamed prostate, BPH, and cancer. Investigations that explain the mechanisms that provide for integrated regulation of cell proliferation, differentiation, and homeostasis will increase our understanding of what goes wrong in the aging prostate, BPH, and prostate cancer. Finally, studies of epithelial and stromal differentiation, together with studies of vascular, neuroendocrine, and neural development provide the tools to identify the epithelial and stromal cell lineages involved in BPH.

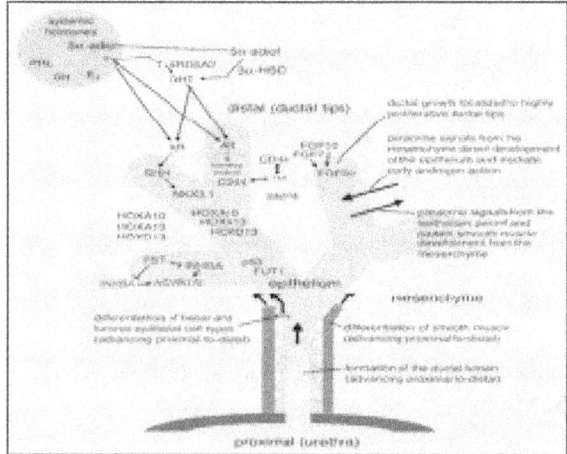

Figure 1. Features of prostatic branching morphogenesis. The diagram shows a generic network of developing prostatic ducts. The developing ductal epithelium is shown in green; the developing prostatic mesenchyme is shown in blue; and the forming ductal lumen is shown in pink. Text annotations indicate general features of prostatic development that have been uncovered by descriptive and experimental embryological studies. Hormones and gene products that have been implicated in prostate development are also shown with developmental expression in epithelium or mesenchyme indicated by the location(s) of the gene or hormone symbol. Factors that act positively to promote growth or morphogenesis of the prostate are shown in black. Factors that act negatively to limit growth or morphogenesis are shown in red.

- Elucidate the mechanisms by which hormonal action, multiple signaling pathways, and transcriptional regulators are integrated to create a complex regulatory program controlling prostate growth and differentiation.
- Assess the role of the extracellular matrix and stromal elements in prostate growth and development. Examine the mechanisms for extracellular matrix regulation.
- Develop validated markers for both epithelial and mesenchymal subpopulations within the developing and adult prostate and use these to define the cell lineages within the prostate.

- Determine the identity and location of stem cell and early progenitor lineages in the developing and adult prostate.
- Characterize the similarities and differences between the rodent and human prostate.
- Determine the mechanisms that regulate the extent of growth during development.
- Examine the role of epigenetics, hormonal, and dietary effects.
- Understand the role of new or incompletely characterized influences on growth during development, including neural and vascular influences; the effect of environmental exposures and diet; and the effect of localized or systemic inflammation.

References:

1. Thomson AA, Marker PC. Branching morphogenesis in the prostate gland and seminal vesicles. *Differentiation* 2006;74(7):382–392.

2. Marker PC, Donjacour AA, Dahiya R, Cunha GR. Hormonal, cellular, and molecular control of prostatic development. *Developmental Biology* 2003;253(2):165–174.

2. Vascular Biology

Angiogenesis is essential to normal physiology and is associated with disease states such as chronic inflammation, arthritis, cancer, and macular degeneration. In the adult, new blood vessels predominantly form from preexisting vasculature via angiogenesis.[1] Angiogenesis inhibition involves sequestration of stimulators of angiogenesis in the extracellular matrix and changes in the endothelial cell shape, reducing their susceptibility to stimulators.[2] Vascular endothelial growth factor (VEGF) is required for vasculature during development.[3]

Normal growth and enlargement of the prostate is regulated by dihydrotestosterone (DHT) and a downstream array of paracrine-acting growth factor signaling cascades. A critical level of androgen is required to maintain prostatic homeostasis and androgen deprivation results in prostatic involution. An intact vascular supply is required to establish and maintain tissue architecture. The extent to which the prostatic vascular system contributes to normal prostate growth control and whether abnormal blood flow patterns in the aging prostate gland lead to hypoxia-stimulated prostate growth is not understood and is in need of further study. A possible relationship between vasculature and homeostasis is suggested by evidence indicating that the prostatic vascular system is a primary androgen action target and that hypoxia elicits cell growth responses.[4] Furthermore,

the contribution of transforming growth factor-β (TGF-β) signaling to prostate homeostasis, in addition to apoptosis, also might involve endothelial cell and myofibroblast response towards neovascularization (Figure 2).[5] This is an important area of study to further define the roles of these factors in prostate growth.

Cardiovascular-active drugs are used for the treatment of obstructive symptoms associated with BPH. Therefore, studying the control of prostate vascularity will substantially enhance our understanding of the etiology of BPH.

Anoikis (cell death upon detachment from extracellular matrix) plays an increasingly recognized key role in angiogenesis.[6] During angiogenesis, cells are in a dynamic state, lacking firm attachment to the extracellular matrix, and exceedingly vulnerable to anoikis. Targeting prostate endothelial cell survival by triggering anoikis may provide a molecular basis for novel prevention strategies for increased prostate vascularity that could contribute to benign and malignant prostate growth. Two classes of angiogenesis-targeting agents with differing modes of action have emerged: (1) those preventing the development of tissue neovasculature (via inducing apoptosis and/or inhibiting cell proliferation and migration); and (2) those that directly target the existing vasculature (via endothelial cell anoikis).[7]

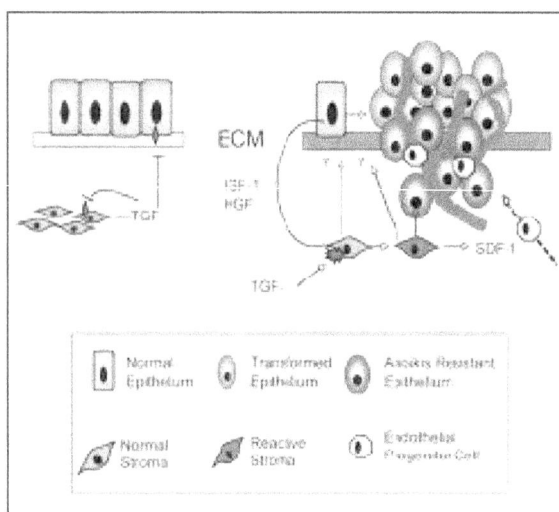

Figure 2. Regulation of prostate vascularity. Prostatic epithelium and stroma are sensitive to TGF-β. The reactive stroma phenotype associated with benign prostate growth involves formation of myofibroblasts, responsible for inducing expression of growth factors such as IGF-1 and HGF contributing to EMT transition of the epithelium. Myofibroblasts induce SDF-1, which attract endothelial progenitor cells towards prostate neovascularization.

- Coordinate genomic and proteomic approaches in human cells and prostate tissues and mouse model systems to establish the role of the vascular system as a regulator of cell survival and the prostate microenvironment.
- Implement studies to understand the crosstalk between endothelial, smooth muscle, and epithelial cell types and regulation by the endocrine system.
- Evaluate the role of hypoxia and inflammation in the context of metabolic syndrome and molecular mechanisms and how this may contribute to benign prostate disease.
- Apply effective new technologies for imaging prostate vascularity to gain insights into integrated neurovascular regulation, regional variations in the vascularity along the ductal axis, and between different zones of the prostate.
- Direct targeting of vessels and endothelial cells within the prostate gland and surrounding organs (e.g., bladder and bladder neck) provides an attractive molecular basis for novel therapeutic strategies for benign prostate diseases.

References:

1. Folkman J. Seminars in medicine of the Beth Israel Hospital, Boston. Clinical applications of research on angiogenesis. *New England Journal of Medicine* 1995;333(26):1757–1763.

2. Risau W. Mechanisms of angiogenesis. *Nature* 1997;386(6626):671–674.

3. Ferrara N, Carver-Moore K, Chen H, et al. Heterozygous embryonic lethality induced by targeted inactivation of the VEGF gene. *Nature* 1996;380(6573):439–442.

4. Ghafar MA, Puchner PJ, Anastasiadis AG, Cabelin MA, Buttyan R. Does the prostatic vascular system contribute to the development of benign prostatic hyperplasia? *Current Urology Reports* 2002;3(4):292–296.

5. Rennebeck G, Martelli M, Kyprianou N. Anoikis and survival connections in the tumor microenvironment: is there a role in prostate cancer metastasis? *Cancer Research* 2005;65(24):11230–11235.

6. Frisch SM, Francis H. Disruption of epithelial cell-matrix interactions induces apoptosis. *Journal of Cell Biology* 1994;124(4):619–626.

7. Ruoslahti E. Antiangiogenics meet nanotechnology. *Cancer Cell* 2002;2(2):97–98.

3. Metabolism

Understanding intermediary metabolism, bioenergetics, and proliferation is highly relevant to benign prostatic diseases. All cells adapt their intermediary metabolism to meet the needs of their differentiated functions.[1] The prostate is distinguished by the accumulation of an extraordinarily high level of citrate acid; prostate secretory epithelial cells have developed specialized mechanisms that involve characteristic alterations in the intermediary metabolism. An associated major metabolic adaptation is the accumulation of a high level of zinc, which inhibits the mitochondrial aconitase reaction and limits citrate oxidation in the Krebs citric acid cycle (Figure 3).[2] As high levels of zinc and citrate are the hallmark of the normal prostate epithelium, the loss of zinc and citrate accumulation is characteristic of prostate cancer.

The specific biological mechanisms of these metabolic alterations and their role in cancer and benign

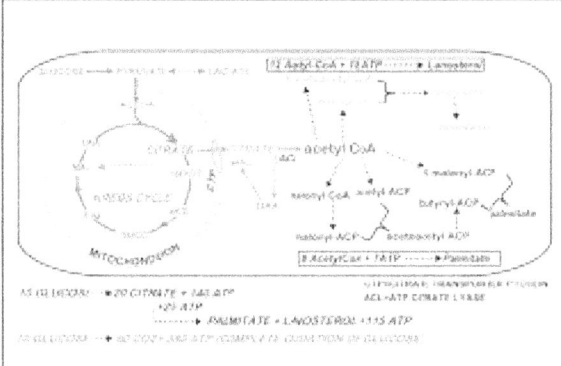

Figure 3. *De novo* lipogenesis/cholesterogenesis begins with the availability of cytosolic acetyl CoA (acetyl CoenzymeA), the common carbon skeleton for fatty acid synthesis (lipogenesis) and for lanesterol synthesis (cholesterogenesis). Therefore, proliferating cells must obtain a source and pathway for cytosolic acetyl CoA synthesis. In mammalian cells, the major source of cytosolic acetyl CoA is derived from the mitochondrial production of citrate, which is exported into the cytosol via a mitochondrial citrate transporter protein (CTP). Normally in mammalian cells CTP expression is low, so that citrate is retained predominantly within the mitochondria, mainly to be oxidized via the Krebs cycle for energy production and also provides intermediates for associated metabolic pathways. Proliferating cells may exhibit an upregulation of CTP, which permits an increased export of citrate to cytosol where it is converted by ATP citrate lyase (ACL) to acetyl CoA + oxalacetate. Thus, in the absence of alternative sources of cytosolic acetyl CoA, proliferating cells must direct their metabolism to optimize mitochondrial production of citrate.

prostatic diseases have not been well studied, but understanding in detail the metabolic transformation that occurs in prostate disease development and its consequences may provide new targets for prostate treatments.

The development and application of metabolomics (i.e., the identification and characterization of small molecules found in an organism) to the normal and the diseased prostate provide a tremendous opportunity to identify metabolic switches and pathway control points that are altered in diseased prostate cell metabolism.

* Encourage studies of changes in intermediary metabolism that accompany inflammation and aging of the prostate.
* Address the effect of the microenvironment on intermediary metabolism through metabolomics.
* Understand the prostate metabolome in the identification of epithelia and stroma cell subpopulation.
* Consider that metabolomics may provide the much-needed assays for the identification of progenitor cells in prostate.
* Investigate the genetic and epigenetic control of gene expression associated with neoplastic and metabolic transformations.

Citrate and zinc are known to decrease in prostate cancer, and detection of citrate by magnetic resonance spectroscopy is already being used to identify foci of prostate cancer *in situ*. In addition, citrate and zinc are increased in BPH, while changes in prostatitic inflammation are being analyzed but remain unclear. These findings suggest that these two factors may have potential as biomarkers for malignant and benign prostate disease.

References:

1. Costello LC, Franklin RB. The intermediary metabolism of the prostate: a key to understanding the pathogenesis and progression of prostate malignancy. *Oncology* 2000;59(4):269–282.

2. Franklin RB, Milon B, Feng P, Costello LC. Zinc and zinc transporters in normal prostate and the pathogenesis of prostate cancer. *Frontiers in Bioscience* 2005;10:2230–2239.

4. Inflammation and Reactive Stroma

Acute inflammation is characterized by a cascade of biochemical events that propagate and mature the inflammatory response, which involves the local vascular system, the immune system, and changes in the stromal cell microenvironment within the injured tissue.[1] Chronic inflammation leads to a progressive shift in the type of cells present at the site of inflammation away from infiltrating neutrophils towards macrophages, lymphocytes, and plasma cells. This process is characterized by simultaneous destruction and healing of the tissue, which involves alterations in the stromal compartment typical of a wound repair response. This may also include recruitment of stem/progenitor cells from either local or circulating populations. A common change in stromal compartment phenotype and physiology (i.e., reactive stroma) is observed in most proliferative disorders in nearly all tissues with an epithelium adjacent to stroma.[2] As the stromal compartment contains vasculature components, nerves, immune components, and fibrous extracellular matrix, it is becoming clear that this compartment is central in any repair process that is initiated in response to tissue damage and loss of tissue homeostasis. Very little is known about the interplay between these processes in the diseased human prostate gland (including BPH and prostatitis) or about the role of growth factors (including cytokines and chemokines), matrix components, and transcription factors—though it is known that mechanisms regulated by these produce proliferative/hyperplastic responses that may or may not accompany inflammation (Figure 4).[3]

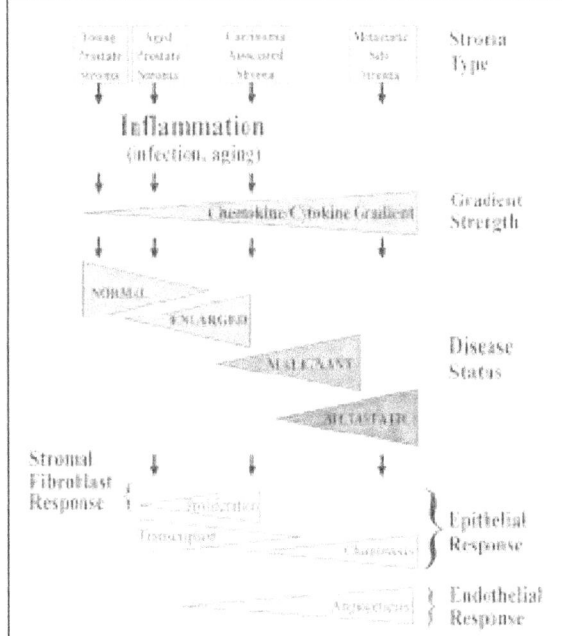

Figure 4. The role of inflammation in prostatic disease. Inflammatory mediators, for example, cytokines and chemokines, secreted at low levels by aging normal-associated prostate stromal fibroblasts and/or consequent to infection, promote the proliferation of both epithelial and stromal fibroblast cell types, as well as gene transcription in epithelial cells, leading to benign prostatic enlargement. Inflammatory mediators secreted by carcinoma-associated fibroblasts facilitate tumor angiogenesis and proliferation, whereas high levels of these mediators secreted by bone marrow stroma comprise a gradient that attracts malignant cells to establish distant metastases.

Inflammatory infiltrate, benign prostatic disease, and reactive stroma changes often coexist in the same prostate.[4] This coexistence can confound attempts to properly diagnose and manage prostatic disease. Development and validation of biomarkers capable of distinguishing prostatic inflammation from benign and malignant prostatic proliferation and prostatitis would provide important diagnostic tools. As an induced stromal reaction is common in most proliferative disorders, including most fibroses, benign growths and premalignant states, targeting such mechanisms as a therapeutic approach is of very high relevance.

Each of the prostate proliferative disease conditions exhibits common features of an induced stromal wound repair type response.[5] This stromal response is pro-repair and therefore pro-proliferation. Such stromal responses are pro-fibrotic as well, and recent evidence shows that these responses are induced very early in proliferative disorders and are likely to be a key to understanding prostate inflammation and how prostate tissue responds to such inflammation. Hence, therapeutic approaches focused on stromal responses, an integral component of stromal-epithelial interactions, and inflammation may be of great use in clinical care at early stages of proliferative prostate diseases.

Research Priorities and Recommendations

There is a need to better understand the causes of prostatic inflammation and associated mechanisms in the healthy and diseased human prostate gland as well as the role they may play in producing a proliferative/ hyperplastic (as is seen in BPH) or prostatitis-type phenotype. In addition, the research priorities for studies of cell-cell (e.g., stromal-epithelial) interactions in prostate disease are multiple. Rodent models are of value to address specific pathways; however, validation in human model systems must be the end-point priority. These studies would be facilitated through examination of multiple *in vitro* and *in vivo* model systems using high-throughput technologies as well as more traditional methods for gene and protein analyses.

The following topics relating to prostate inflammation and the reactive stroma microenvironment are considered novel and important areas for study:

Inflammation:

- Effect of inflammation on prostatic growth.
- The molecular interactions between the various types of immune cells observed in the human prostate (e.g., granulocytes, lymphocytes,

monocytes and macrophages) and prostate epithelial, stromal fibroblast, and endothelial cells need to be examined.

- Mechanisms of immune cell recruitment.
- Role of aging and senescence in inflammation.
- Associated changes in key signaling and homeostatic pathways in response to aging and inflammation.
- Effect of the hormonal milieu on the inflammatory process.
- Effect of prostatic inflammation on bladder function.
- Role of metabolic influences on inflammation.
- Effect of inflammation on neural pathways, sensation, and pain.
- Genetic/racial differences affecting inflammation.
- Animal models of inflammation and injury/repair.
- Role of inflammation in angiogenesis in benign prostatic disease.

Reactive Stroma Microenvironment:

- Conceptual expansion of "stromal-epithelial interactions" to include the interactions with vascular, neural, and inflammatory components.
- Mechanisms of reactive stroma stem/progenitor cell recruitment.
- Stromal-epithelial interactions in the normal prostate and in benign disease.
- Phenotype of reactive stroma associated with benign prostate disease.
- Development of animal models to study the broad array of cell-cell interactions.
- Effects of aging, inflammation, senescence, hormonal changes, and metabolism.
- Alterations of the prostate microenvironment subsequent to inflammation that might facilitate cellular proliferation and/or transformation should be studied.

References:

1. Begley L, Monteleon C, Shah RB, Macdonald JW, Macoska JA. CXCL12 overexpression and secretion by aging fibroblasts enhance human prostate epithelial proliferation *in vitro*. *Aging Cell* 2005;4(6):291–298.

2. Nickel JC, Downey J, Young I, Boag S. Asymptomatic inflammation and/or infection in benign prostatic hyperplasia. *BJU International* 1999;84(9):976–981.

3. Elkahwaji JE, Zhong W, Hopkins WJ, Bushman W. Chronic bacterial infection and inflammation incite reactive hyperplasia in a mouse model of chronic prostatitis. *The Prostate* 2007;67(1):14–21.

4. Tuxhorn JA, Ayala GE, Rowley DR. Reactive stroma in prostate cancer progression. *Journal of Urology* 2001;166(6):2472–2483.

5. Price H, McNeal JE, Stamey TA. Evolving patterns of tissue composition in benign prostatic hyperplasia as a function of specimen size. *Human Pathology* 1990;21(6):578–585.

5. Stem Cells

Stem and early progenitor cells are a critical feature of prostate biology. These have not been thoroughly studied and are likely to play an important role in the response to inflammation, in BPH, and in prostate cancer. Interestingly, stem cells and tumor cells have many common features, including self-renewal, multi-drug resistance, telomerase expression, and, in the case of the prostate, androgen independence. Prostatic stem cells do not require androgens for survival, as evidenced by completely normal prostatic regeneration after multiple cycles of androgen ablation/supplementation.[1]

In the prostate, stem cells are considered to reside in the basal cell compartment (i.e., basal cells are characterized by expression of keratins (CK) 5/14 and the p63 protein). Recent convincing evidence indicates that prostate luminal cells (i.e., fully differentiated epithelial cells) derive from basal cells.[2] As the slow-cycling compartment in the proximal region of murine prostatic ducts is comprised of both basal and luminal cells and as luminal and neuroendocrine cells can develop in the absence of a basal layer, it is possible that luminal cells may have self-renewal properties. Prostate stem cells also have been proposed to contain markers of both basal and luminal cell lineages. In breast epithelium, a bi-potential progenitor that gives rise to both luminal and myoepithelial (basal) cells may reside in the luminal compartment and it is possible a similar bi-potential cell is present in the prostate. Although not well understood, stem/progenitor cells may likely be involved in reactive stroma responses during prostatic hyperplasia/enlargement and prostatitis.

- Identify and characterize stem and progenitor cells for the stromal and epithelial compartments of the normal prostate.
- Determine the lineages and hierarchies in stromal and epithelial compartments as well as characterize their interactions in regulating prostate growth and cellular differentiation.
- Identify prostate-specific markers of both stromal and epithelial progenitors.
- Explore the role of extraprostatic cells in prostate repair and regeneration.
- Consider the study of prostate stem cell biology as a relevant area for assessing congruence between animal model systems and human information databases. This may allow unique connections to be drawn between basic experimental biology and the human prostate in health and disease.

Additional areas of study include:

- The role of the microenvironment and the stem cell niche.
- The effect of inflammation and aging.
- The possibility that BPH is a stem cell disease.
- The role of bladder stem cells in the response to obstruction from an enlarged prostate.
- The distribution of stem cells in rodent and human prostate.
- The sensitivity of stem/progenitor cells to environmental insults and aging.
- The role of the neuroendocrine cell in stem cell biology.

The identification and characterization of prostatic stem cells will likely increase our understanding of normal prostate physiology, but also may lead to new therapeutic approaches for prostate disease, which comprises some of the most common diseases afflicting men.

References:

1. Isaacs JT. Stem cell organization of the prostate and the development of benign prostatic hyperplasia. In: Ackerman R, Schrodder FH, eds. *Prostatic Hyperplasia: Etiology, Surgical and Conservative Management.* Berlin: Walter De Gruyter Inc.; 1989, pp. 23-34.

2. Signoretti S, Pires MM, Lindauer M, et al. p63 regulates commitment to the prostate cell lineage. *Proceedings of the National Academy of Sciences of the United States of America* 2005;102(32):11355–11360.

6. Hormonal Effects

Androgens and estrogens play important roles in prostate homeostasis and development of BPH, though many details of their interplay and effects on key prostate cell types are unclear (Figure 5). In animal models, administration of androgen and estrogen together can cause more dramatic growth stimulation than either alone, arguing that androgens and estrogens act synergistically in the prostate.[1] Changes in androgen and estrogen levels in the aging prostate are likely involved in the development of BPH.[2] Conventional androgen receptor (AR) deletion (i.e., AR knockouts) models have shown that AR is required for prostate development. Tissue recombination and prostate-specific AR deletion studies indicate that AR-stimulated growth is mainly mediated through stromal ARs.[3,4] In addition, deletion of estrogen receptor (ER) sub-type ERα caused a reduction in ductal morphogenesis of the prostate and some ER sub-type ERβ knockout studies argue that ERβ regulates epithelial cellular differentiation.[5] However, several other reports suggest prostates from ERβ knockout mice are normal. Additional studies are clearly needed to obtain a more complete understanding of the hormonal regulation of the prostate.

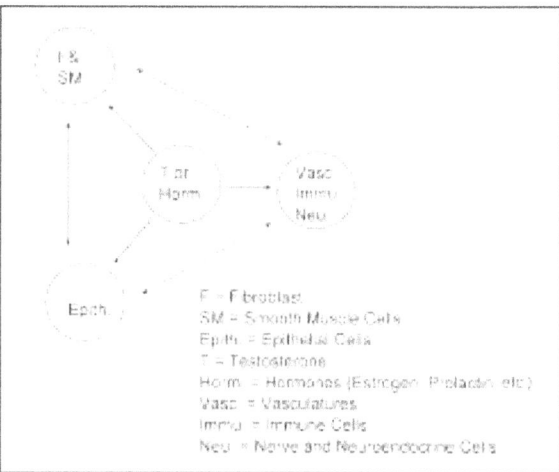

Figure 5. Schematic of interplay between androgen and estrogen hormones on select physiological relevant cell types in the prostate.

- Study the hormonal effects on specific epithelial and stromal progenitor cells and lineages. One important priority is to dissect the cell-specific action of ARs, ERs, retinoic acid receptor, vitamin D receptor, and peroxisome proliferator-activated receptors (PPAR)-gamma. The availability of the murine Cre-lox system allows cell-type specific knockout of AR and/or other steroid receptor genes. Cell-type specific disruption of steroid receptors will provide important insights into the cellular mechanisms of steroid action in the prostate. Genetically modified animals also may be used to validate previous findings regarding the roles of stromal, epithelial, and other cell types in hormone action.

- Investigate the significance of prostate-derived androgens in the overall androgen action. In addition to testosterone and DHT, androgen metabolites also can activate AR and their role in prostate growth should be defined. Recent studies suggest that the prostate can itself produce androgens. One important question is how do androgens affect prostate angiogenesis, vascular integrity, nerves, and immunology?

- Elucidate the regulation of angiogenesis by androgens to provide additional insights into the hormonal regulation of prostate homeostasis. Androgen regulation of prostate vasculature is very dramatic, though the mechanism of this regulation is unclear. Androgens also affect the nervous and immune systems. These effects also are not well defined, particularly at the molecular level, and should be characterized further.

- Characterize specific prostate receptors. Elucidating molecular mechanisms of AR and ER action in the prostate is fundamentally important. Identification and characterization of steroid receptor coregulators and downstream genes may lead to additional targets for modulating hormonal actions in the prostate. Characterization of the regulation of prostate-specific promoters will provide valuable tools for these studies.

- Study the potential crosstalk between androgen- and estrogen-signaling. Androgen-responsive genes and estrogen-responsive genes may influence each other. Identification and characterization of the genes involved in the crosstalk will provide insights into the mechanisms of potential synergy between androgens and estrogen.

- Determine the effect of aging on the hormonal milieu and age-related changes in testosterone and estrogen downstream signaling. Aging is known to affect the hormonal levels in men. The effect of aging on androgen- and/or estrogen-responsive genes in the prostate may represent another important area of research. It is important to investigate whether the effect of aging on hormonally regulated genes in the rodent prostate is similar to that in the human prostate, thus testing its validity as a useful model to study age-related changes in the human prostate. Aging effects on androgen- and/or estrogen-responsive genes in the rodent prostate may provide an opportunity to address molecular mechanisms in BPH development.

- Assess the effect of the hormonal milieu on prostatic inflammation. Hormones can influence prostatic inflammation, which accompanies the production of cytokines and chemokines. The interactions between androgens and inflammatory pathways may play important roles in BPH development.

- Assess the roles of prolactin in the prostate. Prolactin is another hormone important in prostate growth. The involvement of prolactin in BPH will need to be fully investigated.

- Address possible neuroendocrine effects. Neurendocrine secretions may influence prostate growth and function. Therefore, studies in this area should be considered.

- Work to understand how changes in the levels of androgens, estradiol, prolactin, and other hormones may be causative factors in BPH. Changes in hormone levels may lead to abnormal expression of some key hormone responsive genes, resulting in disruption of normal prostatic homeostasis. Identification of the key hormonally regulated genes may provide novel targets for prevention and treatment of BPH.

References:

1. Walsh PC, Wilson JD. The induction of prostatic hypertrophy in the dog with androstanediol. *Journal of Clinical Investigation* 1976;57(4):1093–1097.

2. Leav I, Merk FB, Kwan PW, Ho SM. Androgen-supported estrogen-enhanced epithelial proliferation in the prostates of intact Noble rats. *The Prostate* 1989;15(1):23–40.

References (continued):

3. Sugimura Y, Cunha GR, Bigsby RM. Androgenic induction of DNA synthesis in prostatic glands induced in the urothelium of testicular feminized (Tfm/Y) mice. *The Prostate* 1986;9(3):217–225.

4. Simanainen U, Allan CM, Lim P, et al. Disruption of prostate epithelial androgen receptor impedes prostate lobe-specific growth and function. *Endocrinology* 2007;148(5):2264–2272.

5. Jarred RA, McPherson SJ, Bianco JJ, Couse JF, Korach KS, Risbridger GP. Prostate phenotypes in estrogen-modulated transgenic mice. *Trends in Endocrinology and Metabolism TEM* 2002;13(4):163–168.

7. Animal Models

Progress in understanding and treating human urological diseases is absolutely dependent on adequate animal models. Concentrating efforts to create mouse models allows researchers to take advantage of the extensive knowledge of mouse genetics, as well as the numerous knockout and conditional mice that already exist. Genetically Engineered Mouse (GEM) models would allow for specific manipulation of genes implicated in prostatitis and BPH. The goal here is to create mouse lesions that closely resemble human disease in terms of pathology, molecular alterations that accompany progression, and behavior (such as the ability of BPH to locally cause urethra obstruction). Adequacy of murine models can be optimized by basing the nature of the genetic/molecular manipulation on pathways identified as involved in human prostate disease. Unfortunately, our understanding of the molecular pathways involved in prostatitis and BPH are very limited. Therefore, making GEM models to the pathways responsible for human prostate diseases may be difficult. However, it is currently possible to develop models that demonstrate features of human disorders, particularly in terms of histology and symptoms.

BPH is considered to be a disease not simply of epithelial overgrowth but also of stromal overgrowth. Currently, there is no promoter that can be used to target genes in prostatic stroma. Furthermore, mouse models for prostate cancer have demonstrated that stromal proliferation occurs even though stromal cells were not directly targeted by the epithelial cell-specific promoter. This suggests a crosstalk between the epithelium and stroma, which returns us to the role of the microenvironment during the disease process. Despite such hurdles, experience in making prostate cancer models demonstrates the feasibility of making the models for BPH.[1]

Developing new rodent models for benign prostate disease would expand our ability to test therapeutic treatment during the disease processes and methods to relieve symptoms after the urologic disorder is established. Mouse models for cancer have become sources to develop new cell lines that can be used either for *in vitro* studies or regrafted in hosts to create allograft models. If this also held true for new models of benign disease, it would be of great use to the community.

Research Priorities and Recommendations

Research on prostatitis and BPH is greatly limited by the lack of adequate models for these urologic diseases. One serious roadblock to creating new GEM (or rat) models for BPH is our inability to specifically target prostatic stroma.

The following priorities exist:

* Create new models, potentially by examining existing mouse models in which the transgene has been targeted to the prostatic epithelium or null mice to determine if any are appropriate to model prostatitis or BPH.
* Develop new approaches to target prostatic stroma with the goal of developing new GEM (or rat) models. Once new models are developed, further tools such as methods to image pathology and to follow therapeutic intervention with tissue-specific reporters will be needed. Also, mouse models that already exist and have different cell types tagged with imaging markers may be useful for imaging and following biological changes during development of disease and therapeutic intervention.
* Standardize analysis of the GEM models to ensure that phenotypic changes that occur are correctly defined from model to model.
* Provide mouse models reflecting prostatitis and BPH to determine pathways relevant to the diseases and to establish therapeutic models for testing new drugs.

References:

1. Shappell SB, Thomas GV, Roberts RL, et al. Prostate pathology of genetically engineered mice: definitions and classification. The consensus report from the Bar Harbor meeting of the Mouse Models of Human Cancer Consortium Prostate Pathology Committee. *Cancer Research* 2004;64(6):2270–2305.

8. Aging

Benign prostate disease and prostate cancer are among the most commonly diagnosed diseases in the male U.S. population. Several etiological factors including aging and diet have been strongly implicated in the development of these diseases.[1,2,3] How these factors contribute to the initiation and progression at the molecular level remains elusive. In addition, studies have demonstrated an accumulation of somatic mutations that generate oxidative damage in the aging prostate, thus suggesting a role in disease development. These relationships also remain unclear. Interestingly, similar mechanisms may be present in pelvic organs besides the prostate, such as the bladder and urethra.

There is growing recent interest in the role of epigenetics (i.e., changes in chromatin or DNA modification that do not involve changes in DNA sequence) in disease susceptibility during aging. For example, global DNA hypomethylation occurs in the prostate with aging.[4] Also, of potential relevance, focal hypermethylation has been found in the aging colon at several loci, including the IGF2 promoter and estrogen receptor. Such changes may alter growth regulation in benign prostate disease and prostate cancer. In the case of prostate cancer, it is clear that the "normal" tissue surrounding the cancer lesions display a number of molecular changes that are potentially age related.[5] Array work has identified specific changes that occur with the development of benign prostate disease (e.g., BPH).[6,7,8] One unique aspect of epigenetic changes is that they are reversible. Furthermore, they may be modulated by the environment.[9] In addition, diet, oxidative stress, and other factors may affect epigenetic changes.[10]

Research Priorities and Recommendations

Given the strong link between BPH (and prostate cancer) and aging, this area provides fertile ground for new research. In addition, it is likely that data generated will have applicability to other diseases associated with aging (e.g., colon and breast cancer).

Opportunities for research include:

- Identify histopathologic changes in rodent and human prostate and other urogenital tissues that occur with aging.
- Determine the impact of senescence and senescence cells on the development of benign prostate disease (e.g., BPH), prostate cancer, and other urologic diseases. Furthermore, study whether or not the occurrence of senescence is obligatorily with aging.
- Identify epigenetic changes in human urogenital tissues with aging. These include DNA methylation changes, alterations in histone modifications, changes in genomic imprinting, and others. Also, study the effect of inflammation and other factors associated with aging on epigenetic processes.
- Assess the link between epigenetic changes that occur with aging in the prostate and the development of prostate disease, and if they may predict disease outcomes.
- Evaluate the potential for these changes to be reversible or preventable.
- Study additional unknowns regarding aging and epigenetics, including the influence of hormones, genetic and racial differences, and whether there is a response to prostatitis. In addition, identify epigenetic changes in the bladder in response to obstruction.

References:

1. Kwabi-Addo B, Chung W, Shen L, et al. Age-related DNA methylation changes in normal human prostate tissues. *Clinical Cancer Research* 2007;13(13):3796–3802.

2. Malins DC, Johnson PM, Wheeler TM, Barker EA, Polissar NL, Vinson MA. Age-related radical-induced DNA damage is linked to prostate cancer. *Cancer Research* 2001;61(16):6025–6028.

3. Atwood CS, Barzilai N, Bowen RL, et al. Pennington scientific symposium on mechanisms and retardation of aging. *Experimental Gerontology* 2003;38(10):1217–1226.

References (continued):

4. Bennett-Baker PE, Wilkowski J, Burke DT. Age-associated activation of epigenetically repressed genes in the mouse. *Genetics* 2003;165(4):2055–2062.

5. Campisi J. Aging and cancer: the double-edged sword of replicative senescence. *Journal of the American Geriatrics Society* 1997;45(4):482–488.

6. Chang BD, Watanabe K, Broude EV, et al. Effects of p21Waf1/Cip1/Sdi1 on cellular gene expression: implications for carcinogenesis, senescence, and age-related diseases. *Proceedings of the National Academy of Sciences of the United States of America* 2000;97(8):4291–4296.

7. Dimri GP, Lee X, Basile G, et al. A biomarker that identifies senescent human cells in culture and in aging skin *in vivo*. *Proceedings of the National Academy of Sciences of the United States of America* 1995;92(20):9363–9367.

8. Fu VX, Schwarze SR, Kenowski ML, Leblanc S, Svaren J, Jarrard DF. A loss of insulin-like growth factor-2 imprinting is modulated by CCCTC-binding factor down-regulation at senescence in human epithelial cells. *Journal of Biological Chemistry* 2004;279(50):52218–52226.

9. Jaenisch R, Bird A. Epigenetic regulation of gene expression: how the genome integrates intrinsic and environmental signals. *Nature Genetics* 2003;33(Suppl):245–254.

10. Mathers JC. Nutritional modulation of ageing: genomic and epigenetic approaches. *Mechanisms of Ageing and Development* 2006;127(6):584–589.

9. Signaling

Information flow within cells and between cellular and tissue compartments occurs in part through signaling pathways, which are characterized by a complex web of biochemical processes involving a myriad of synchronized events at the protein level. Biochemical steps in such signaling pathways may include post-translational modifications of newly synthesized proteins, such as phosphorylation, palmitoylation, and sumoylation; interactions between kinases and non-enzymatic proteins, such as protein adapters and scaffolds; sequestration within specialized subcellular compartments; regulated cleavage by proteinases; intracellular transport; regulated secretion into the extracellular space; assembly, stabilization, and disassembly of large, multimeric signaling complexes; and ubiquitination and proteasome-mediated degradation. Most of these events are capable of providing critical regulatory control over cell growth, cell survival and programmed cell death, neovascularization/angiogenesis, and membrane structure and trafficking.[1] An emerging area of interest is the control of lipid-dependent events in cell signaling.[2] Many of these basic processes are understood in biochemical terms and have been described in some detail (an example of such a signaling pathway for communicating signals from the cell surface to intracellular signaling components is depicted in Figure 6). However, there are enormous gaps in our knowledge, particularly with respect to cellular signaling in clinical pathologies seen in human disease, including benign disease of the prostate.

Research Priorities and Recommendations

Most cell and tissue-specific signal transduction mechanisms relevant to the adult human prostate and benign prostatic disease are poorly understood and characterized. The male urogenital tract is an organ system that demonstrates pronounced age-dependent changes, as well as "inflammatory" events in young individuals that are not well understood. In most cases, the biochemical events and pathways underlying and possibly causing these changes are unknown. The effect of aging on signaling pathway function and integration and the extent to which changes in inflammatory signaling cascades intersect with non-pathophysiologic, age-dependent changes remain unknown.

Rapid progress in this area relies on providing the following resources:

* Improved basic knowledge about signaling webs.
* Powerful new bioinformatics tools and databases infrastructure leading to knowledge of the functional roles of proteins and protein modifications in various signaling processes.
* New reagents and imaging tools that allow analyses of cellular and tissue signaling events with high resolution in intact animals.
* Widespread use of invertebrate and lower vertebrate model systems that allow a high level of functional assessment of proteins and signaling pathways.

- Mass spectrometric techniques that permit extensive analysis and characterization of multiprotein complexes and protein modifications on a large scale (e.g., the comprehensive identification of every phosphorylation site of a large protein in one or a few experiments).
- Unprecedented opportunities for crossfertilization exist between disciplines at technical and conceptual levels in the study of prostate signaling events.

The potential contributions of signal transduction research to the clinical setting in the context of benign prostate disease lie principally in two arenas:

1) Elucidation of disease-relevant pathways, proteins, and biochemical events, opening the way for application of targeted therapy based on known physiological mechanisms.

2) Identification of disease biomarkers that allow proper diagnosis, disease categorization, and clinically relevant prognostic information.

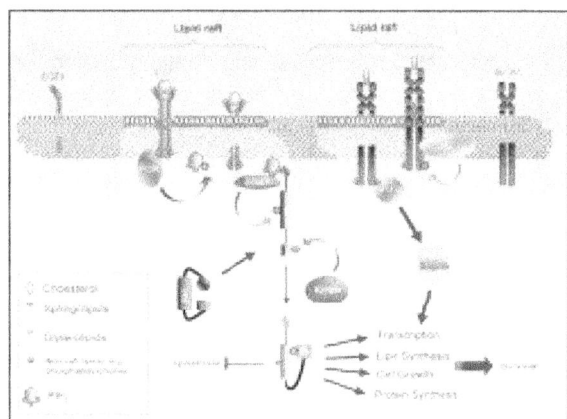

Figure 8. Crosstalk between signal transduction pathways regulated in part by association of one or more signaling intermediates with cholesterol- and sphingolipid-enriched microdomains, known as lipid rafts.[2]

References:

1. Cohen AW, Hnasko R, Schubert W, Lisanti MP. Role of caveolae and caveolins in health and disease. *Physiological Reviews* 2004;84(4):1341–1379.

2. Hager MH, Solomon KR, Freeman MR. The role of cholesterol in prostate cancer. *Current Opinion in Clinical Nutrition and Metabolic Care* 2006;9(4):379–385.

10. Neurobiology

The prostate receives abundant innervation from both the sympathetic and parasympathetic neuronal pathways. The predominant adrenergic input to the prostate, as well as to other male internal genitalia, is from the short adrenergic neurons located near the prostate and from the sympathetic chain.[1,2] Pharmacological studies have shown that adrenergic innervation elicits smooth muscle contraction and cholinergic innervation evokes glandular secretion. Prostatic sensory nerves have been identified, but their functional role is unclear. Contractile and secretory activities are dependent on an intact nerve supply for normal functioning of the prostate.[3] In addition, neural innervation exerts a trophic control on prostatic tissue.

Neural peptides, including vasoactive intestinal polypeptides (VIP), enkephalins, and neuropeptide Y (NPY), have been identified in prostate nerve fibers, but their role has not yet been identified. The role of nitric oxide (NO) as a regulator of prostatic secretion and excretion has been described recently, but its functional significance is not clear. Catecholamines can function as mitogens in several target tissues, including the prostate gland, acting directly through the adrenergic receptors or through receptor-mediated induction of other growth factors, such as epithelial growth factor (EGF). Catecholamines alone or in conjunction with androgens may, therefore, be important physiologic regulators of the human prostate gland. Recently, studies demonstrated increased levels of apoptosis in human prostate specimens from men who were treated with alpha-1 antagonists. The possible role of adrenergic activity in hyperplasia has not been adequately investigated.

The prostate, as well as the prostatic urethra, contains numerous neuroendocrine cells located in the ductal epithelium. These cells stain positively for serotonin, as well as a variety of peptides, and display microvilli extending into the ductal lumen. Their morphology is extremely similar to gastrointestinal enteroendocrine cells and strongly suggests a chemosensory function, though their true function remains to be described.

Prostatic neuroendocrine cells have been implicated in promotion of both benign and cancerous prostatic growth and their study remains an area demanding more intensive investigation.[4,5] The previously demonstrated effects of sympathectomy and parasympathectomy on prostate growth regulation support the conclusion that the dichotomy of function in ventral prostate autonomic innervation is real and has a fundamental regulatory purpose.[6] Finding the mechanism of contralateral hyperplasia and ipsilateral atrophy has potential significance in the investigation and understanding of abnormal human prostatic growth.

Research Priorities and Recommendations

Experimental studies indicate that neural manipulations can exert significant control over prostate growth. There is an urgent need to identify the mechanisms by which innervation regulates growth.

Specific areas of recommended focus include:

- Assess abnormal innervation of the pelvic floor as a possible underlying contributor to benign disorders of the prostate (e.g., such as those involving pelvic pain as a symptom).
- Conduct experimental animal studies and studies on human tissues to identify changes in prostate innervation with aging, metabolic syndrome, and diabetes.
- Encourage studies of the role of sensory innervation in health and disease, especially as it relates to urologic pelvic pain.
- Foster studies to determine if age- or disease-related neuronal alterations underlie benign prostate disease.
- Analyze the role of the nitric oxide system in the prostate. Pathophysiological changes in this system and their role in abnormal prostatic growth needs to be determined.
- Investigate the mechanism of action of PDE5 inhibitors in BPH/LUTS in animal and human studies.
- Conduct characterization of prostate serotonergic neuroendocrine cells. Also, examine the role of these cells in pathological growth.
- Identify the environmental factors affecting prostatic function (e.g., endocrine, circadian, dietary factors).

References:

1. Abrahamsson PA, di Sant'Agnese PA. Neuroendocrine cells in the human prostate gland. *Journal of Andrology* 1993;14(5):307–309.

2. McVary KT, McKenna KE, Lee C. Prostate innervation. *The Prostate Supplement* 1998;8:2–13.

3. Haynes JM, Ventura S. Current models of human prostate contractility. *Clinical and Experimental Pharmacology & Physiology* 2005;32(10):797–804.

4. Noordzij MA, van Steenbrugge GJ, van der Kwast TH, Schroder FH. Neuroendocrine cells in the normal, hyperplastic and neoplastic prostate. *Urological Research* 1995;22(6):333–341.

5. McVary KT, Rademaker A, Lloyd GL, Gann P. Autonomic nervous system overactivity in men with lower urinary tract symptoms secondary to benign prostatic hyperplasia. *Journal of Urology* 2005;174(4 Pt 1):1327–1433.

6. Santamaria L, Ingelmo I, Alonso L, Pozuelo JM, Rodriguez R. Neuroendocrine cells and peptidergic innervation in human and rat prostate. *Advances in Anatomy, Embryology, and Cell Biology* 2007;194:1–77.

11. Proteomics and New Technologies

Although genomic data and transcript profiling offer tremendous opportunities to identify and understand molecular alterations in disease, even the complete "genetic blueprint" has serious limitations. Apart from the obvious fact that cellular functions are carried out by proteins, not by DNA and RNA, there are numerous protein modifications that are not apparent from the nucleic acid or amino acid sequence. These include differential RNA splicing and post-translational modifications such as phosphorylation and glycosylation. In addition, the genomic sequence does not specify which proteins interact, how interactions occur, or where in the cell a protein localizes under various conditions. Moreover, transcript abundance levels do not always correlate with protein abundance levels and one cannot tell from the genomic sequence whether a gene is ever translated into protein or rather functions as RNA.

Recent genetic triumphs have been paralleled by a surge in interest in the comprehensive study of proteins and protein systems. This field has been dubbed "proteomics," a word derived from proteome, meaning the complete set of proteins expressed by the genome. From a biomedical standpoint, the field of proteomics has great potential, as the bulk of pharmacological interventions and diagnostic tests are directed at proteins rather than genes. The inherent advantage afforded to proteomics over genomics is that the identified protein is itself the biological end product.

The behavior of proteins is determined by the tertiary structure of the molecule. Any assay based on protein binding depends on maintaining the native conformation of the protein. This puts constraints on the systems used to capture protein targets in affinity-based assays. Second, the detection of low-abundance proteins poses a particular challenge, especially given that the dynamic ranges of proteins in biological systems can reach parts per million or greater. An amplification system analogous to the polymerase chain reaction has yet to be developed for protein studies. In addition, the behavior of proteins may or may not be governed quantitatively. Protein regulation is often based not on synthesis and degradation, but on reversible modifications (e.g., phosphorylation). Adding to the complexity is that RNA splicing may produce splice variants that are highly homologous though differ in function. Nonetheless, protein science has advanced to the point that some of these hurdles can be overcome.

Until recently, the study of global protein expression was performed nearly exclusively using two-dimensional gel electrophoresis. This technique allows the display of thousands of proteins as spots on a rectangular gel, though it is somewhat cumbersome, labor intensive, insensitive, and not suitable for high-throughput applications. Due to these limitations, new approaches for performing large-scale protein studies have been developed that include mass spectrometry, yeast two-hybrid systems, and protein arrays. Application of proteomics to the study of genitourinary biology, including study of the prostate, is an emerging discipline. The potential applications of proteomics-based approaches mandate that the technologies in the early phases of development be applied to important problems in the field of prostate biology and pathology.

Emphasizing priorities for proteomics is inherently distinct from hypothesis-driven questions, as this area is generally technology driven.

The following recommendations will facilitate the development/application of new technologies to the study of benign prostate disorders:

- Develop and validate quantitative methods for comprehensive measurements of protein abundance levels in complex mixtures (e.g., tissue/body fluids). Absolute quantitation is ideal, but relative quantitation also would be quite useful. Such approaches are still poorly standardized and rarely cross-compared (e.g., isotope-coded affinity tag, "Shotgun" approaches, stable isotope labeling of amino acids in cell culture, anti-peptide antibodies, etc.).
- Develop standards for data reporting and data deposition analogous to Minimum Information About a Microarray Experiment standards for microarray experiments. Develop archives/databases to house proteomics data (e.g., analogous to the Gene Expression Omnibus).
- Develop methods for exploring the low abundance proteome and for comprehensive analyses of post-translational protein modifications and spatial relationships/integrity of cell types and microenvironment molecules.
- Focus on integrated disease-related studies involving analyses of protein complexes (extracted and preserved intact) to detail the assembly of molecules necessary for specific biological function (e.g., the complex of co-regulatory factors involved with AR activation or repression).
- Develop a program integrating proteomic and metabolomic analysis to investigate the unique metabolism of the prostate and potential changes due to infection, aging, and/or inflammation.
- Develop in vitro imaging systems to investigate modifications and interactions between multiple proteins simultaneously. In vitro imaging systems also would be useful if applied to the real-time analysis of a single cell.
- Disseminate bioinformatics tools capable of integrating data from profiles of transcripts, proteins, and post-translational protein modifications.

- Develop "network-based" analysis tools that incorporate experimental datasets and individual laboratory experiments (e.g., Ingenuity, Cytoscape, etc.).

Establishing new approaches and standards for the comprehensive (or at a minimum, high-throughput) measurement of multiple protein/protein modifications has the potential to impact essentially every area of emphasis involving prostatic diseases. These methods could assist with basic laboratory-based studies of disease pathogenesis and also inform clinical studies of risk, treatment-response, and host-pathogen interaction. A key future focus involves concepts relating to personalized medicine, assessments of biomarkers of disease, and integration with biomedical imaging (e.g., proteins serve as the optimal scaffolds for directing tissue/cell-specific imaging probes).

Related research priorities include:

- Establish a reference database for the normal variation of protein abundance, protein isoforms, and protein modifications in the prostate (human and rodent). Databases detailing such variability at the transcript level have greatly facilitated array-based studies of gene expression changes associated with other diseases. In addition, resulting data could be integrated with transcript profiles and with SNP-based studies of human variation.
- Determine which—and to what extent—protein levels (and modifications) change as a result of surgical resection of the prostate; prostate biopsy; and prostate tissue sample fixation/freezing and storage.
- Support an in-depth analysis of prostatic secretome (i.e., prostate-derived secretory products in seminal fluid or plasma) to facilitate studies of changes associated with infectious or inflammatory diseases.

12. Infrastructure Needs

Human Tissue

Human tissues of various types and from various patient ages are needed for the examination of BPH and other prostate diseases. Improved availability of human fetal prostate tissue is a key need for the study of human prostate development. With regard to adult prostate tissues, a shift in the technique of acquisition has occurred with the advent of laparoscopic robotic prostatectomy. Roughly 25 percent of prostate specimens will be removed via this approach in 2006 versus the standard open approach and this is likely to increase over time. This procedure entails additional warm ischemia time (30–60 minutes) prior to specimen removal from the body. Labile proteins, enzymes, and some RNA components will likely be altered with this approach to a greater extent than with open prostatectomy. These aspects need to be considered when judging research studies, and highlight the need for validation of specimens prior to their use in research. Continued funding and development of centralized tissue resources with open access is a high priority.

Interdisciplinary Research

There is growing evidence that benign prostate diseases occur in parallel with other organ-specific diseases and systemic conditions, including metabolic syndrome, cardiovascular disease, diabetes, and erectile dysfunction. These connections are being explored at a clinical level. However, there is a compelling need to promote interdisciplinary research focusing on mechanisms linking these conditions.

There is a great need for focus on hypothesis generation, discovery, and infrastructure development that do not require a specific research hypothesis. Appropriate funding mechanisms should be used that call for the achievement of specific milestones to ensure continued progress in the field.

Training and Fellowship Programs

Training programs that encourage young investigators to pursue careers in benign prostate research are important for future development in the field. These efforts would be aided by increasing the visibility and recognition of this research—something that might be most effectively communicated by promoting interdisciplinary research and developing a high-profile scientific venue (e.g., a prostate research-specific Gordon Conference). There should be a special effort to bring together independent basic scientists and clinical fellows and junior faculty to develop collaborative and bidirectional research efforts. Increasing fellowship funding opportunities are recommended for urologists to pursue basic science training and to create mechanisms that require collaborations between urologists, clinicians from other disciplines, and basic scientists.

We recognize the need for incentives for talented science and math students to go into prostate basic research and applied research using molecular approaches; incentives for clinicians to stay involved in biomedical research; and the need to overcome perceived and objective barriers between long-term collaborative relationships between chemists, biophysicists, molecular biologists, and clinical scientists.

New Meeting Venue

There is a need to elevate the visibility of prostate biology and lower urinary tract disease research. A strong recommendation is to establish a Gordon Conference focused on prostate biology and benign lower urinary tract diseases.

High-Priority Recommendations

Both clinically defined BPH and prostatitis often involve changes in bladder function, pelvic floor function, neuronal function, and may coexist with other systemic conditions. These associated conditions may be as important as the changes occurring in the prostate, therefore calling for the development of new clinical paradigms and comprehensive research approaches.

The major, targeted priorities for benign prostate disease basic research are the following:

* Create new models for the study of benign prostate disease.
* Develop a comprehensive understanding of the signaling, interaction, and crosstalk between multiple cell-types in the prostate.

* Understand the effect of aging on prostate biology and lower urogenital system function.
* Apply new technologies and imaging techniques.
* Diversify efforts to establish points of biological congruence between cell and animal models and the human prostate that will facilitate translational research.
* Characterize disease-relevant cellular pathways to open the way for application of "smart" (i.e., targeted) therapies based on known physiological mechanisms.
* Encourage an integrated and multifaceted study of endocrine regulation of lower urogenital biology.
* Promote training and career development efforts for investigators interested in research careers in benign prostate disease.

II. Epidemiology/ Population-Based Studies

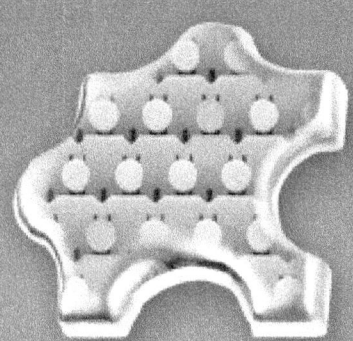

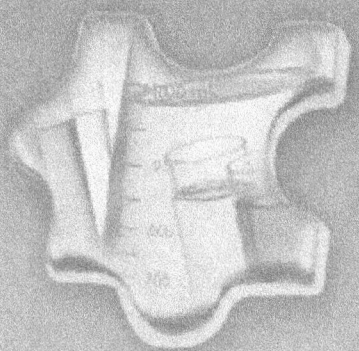

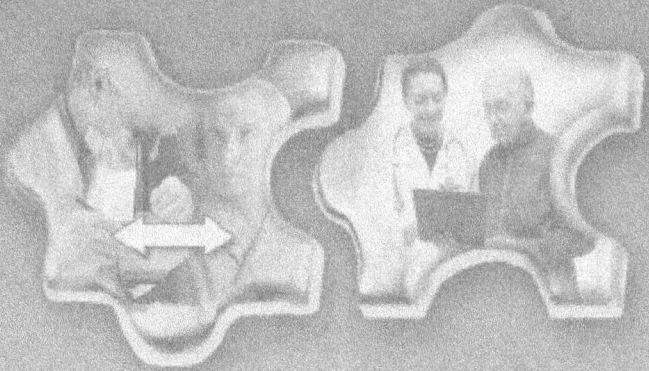

Mission Statement

The central mission of the Epidemiology/Population-Based Studies section is to promote the use of epidemiological and population-based sciences and health services research in multidisciplinary teams to better translate knowledge between the community, the clinic, and the laboratory. This is anticipated to improve our understanding of disease etiology, management, and outcomes for benign prostate disease.

Epidemiology and health services research play a critical role in advancing the goal of biomedical research in improving the health of the population. Application of epidemiologic and health services methods is necessary to translate basic research findings into more effective disease prevention strategies, enhance clinical practice, and improve education and knowledge dissemination. Indeed, epidemiologic and health services research methods are central for the design, analysis, and translation of both basic and clinical research studies.

A key impediment to progress in this field is the lack of standard definitions for benign prostatic diseases. Also, epidemiologic and health services studies have not been successful in identifying risk factors that are amenable to prevention. To address these issues, population scientists will have to partner with basic and clinical scientists to change the existing paradigms and develop disease classifications based on etiology. Insights generated from the laboratory bench, integrated physiology studies, and clinical and population-based research will be required to develop a more meaningful classification system. Without such actions, continued progress in this area will be hindered.

pidemiology is defined as a branch of medical science that deals with occurrence, distribution, and disease control in a population. This area of research is very important for understanding aspects of benign prostate disease, such as benign prostatic hyperplasia (BPH), or enlargement of the prostate, and chronic pain conditions often associated with the prostate-like chronic prostatitis. Research in large populations of individuals and research focused on health care delivery are critical areas of investigation and are complementary to basic science research and clinical trials. Research findings in these areas help to identify risk factors for disease development or progression, create standards for measuring disease severity, and address questions about how best to optimize clinical care for patients. Accordingly, this section emphasizes the need to expand current research efforts to better emphasize epidemiology, patterns of care, quality of care, cost studies, and decision making. Also, collaborations between researchers who understand scientific methods and clinicians who provide care for benign prostate disease are required, as research in the absence of clinical relevance will not improve care.

Scientific Topics/Areas of Research

13. Epidemiology of Prostatitis

The study of the epidemiology of prostatitis is hampered by the fact that what is commonly referred to as prostatitis actually comprises four different conditions:

Category I. Acute bacterial prostatitis, which is associated with symptoms of bacterial infection.

Category II. Chronic bacterial prostatitis, which is caused by a chronic bacterial infection of the prostate with or without symptoms of infection.

Category III. Chronic prostatitis/chronic pelvic pain syndrome (CP/CPPS), which is characterized by pelvic pain, possible voiding symptoms, and a lack of apparent infection.

Category IV. Asymptomatic inflammatory prostatitis, which is characterized by evidence of prostate inflammation, but an absence of symptoms.

Furthermore, these various conditions often occur in men under the age of 65. Therefore, many existing databases that are available for epidemiologic analysis (e.g., Medicare) have limited relevance to the study of prostatitis. Insights into the epidemiology of prostatitis and some existing limitations are described in the paragraphs that follow.

Prevalence

Prevalence is generally defined as the degree to which the percentage of a population is affected with a particular disease at a given time. The prevalence of prostatitis (Figure 1) has been previously assessed through five means:

1) Prevalence of histologic inflammation at autopsy. This has limited clinical relevance.
2) Prevalence of self-reported prostatitis. This is subject to recall bias. Prevalence estimates have ranged from 14 to 16 percent.
3) Prevalence of prostatitis-like symptoms. This is subject to response bias, as individuals with symptoms may be more likely to participate than those without symptoms. Prevalence estimates have ranged from 2.7 to 9.7 percent. Of note, one study in Malaysia included a clinical evaluation of a subgroup of the men identified with prostatitis-like symptoms.[1] In their population, 8.7 percent of men exhibited prostatitis symptoms. In the subgroup of men who were examined, 75 percent met the clinical criteria for CP/CPPS.
4) Prevalence of physician-diagnosed prostatitis. This identifies a rather heterogeneous group that comprises men with all four types of prostatitis, plus men with brief, self-limited symptoms such as dysuria (i.e., painful urination) who are diagnosed with "prostatitis" for lack of a better explanation

for the symptoms. Prevalence estimates have ranged from 4.5 to 9 percent.

5) Number of yearly physician visits for prostatitis. This does not yield a prevalence estimate, as we do not know how many patients had multiple visits. Also, as stated in number 4 above, this method identifies a heterogeneous group of individuals. According to National Ambulatory Medical Care Survey (NAMCS) data, in 2000 there were 1,795,643 physician office visits with prostatitis listed as any diagnosis, which yielded a rate of 1,867 per 100,000.[2]

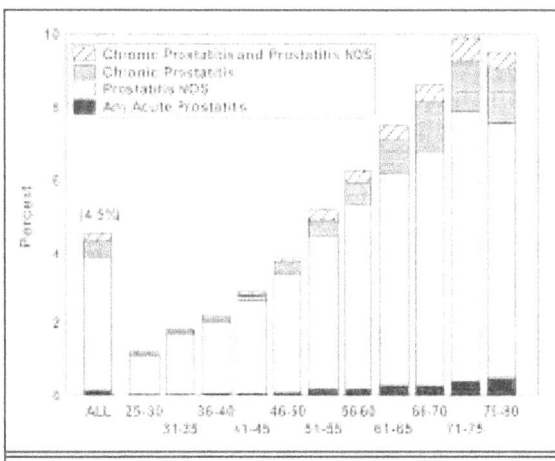

Figure 1. Age-specific prevalence of physician-diagnosed prostatitis in Kaiser Permanante Northwest.[6]

Incidence

Incidence is generally defined as the rate of occurrence or influence. Unlike prevalence, incidence studies of prostatitis are uncommon and have used medical record review to confirm diagnosis. In Olmsted County, Minnesota, the incidence rates were 3.1/1000 person-years for all types of prostatitis, 2.8/1000 person-years for acute prostatitis, and 0.7/1000 person-years for chronic prostatitis. In the Kaiser Permanente Northwest (Portland, Oregon) managed care population, the incidence was 4.9/1000 person-years for all types of prostatitis, and 3.3/1000 person-years for category III prostatitis.[3]

Natural History

The natural history of prostatitis (i.e., progression of disease) has not been completely studied. The low prevalence of category I and category II prostatitis makes it difficult and perhaps impossible to study the natural history of these conditions. The natural history of category IV prostatitis is an area of considerable research interest (e.g., the relationship between inflammation and prostate cancer or BPH). There are very little data regarding the natural history of category III prostatitis despite the significant clinical relevance of this issue. In the NIH-Chronic Prostatitis Cohort Study, 293 men with CP/CPPS were followed for 2 years.[4] There was a slight improvement in mean NIH-Chronic Prostatitis Symptom Index (NIH-CPSI) scores over this interval, and approximately one-third exhibited moderate or marked improvement in symptoms. No demographic or clinical factors were identified that predicted symptoms change over time.

Risk Factors/Comorbidities

Although the etiology and to a large degree the pathogenesis of CP/CPPS (i.e., non-bacterial, chronic, category III prostatitis) are unknown, existing epidemiologic data provide some clues. Infection is commonly cited as a possible cause for CP/CPPS. In the NIDDK-sponsored Chronic Prostatitis Clinical Research Network (CPCRN) study, cases and controls did not differ in age, education, employment status, or sexual history, but cases reported a significantly greater lifetime prevalence of non-specific urethritis (i.e., inflammation of the urethra). This is consistent with a study of more than 30,000 males in which men reporting a history of sexually transmitted disease had 1.8-fold greater odds of a self-reported history of prostatitis.

In the CPCRN study, cases were significantly more likely to report additional disorders.[5] This included a six times greater incidence of cardiovascular disease, which was predominantly hypertension. In addition, cases reported a five times greater history of neurologic disease and a 2.5 times greater history of psychiatric disease. Hematopoietic, lymphatic, or infectious disease, specifically sinusitis, was twice as common in the cases as controls. One study using the Kaiser Permanente Northwest database found that men with prostatitis were more likely to be diagnosed with other urologic conditions, unexplained somatic symptoms, and psychiatric conditions.[6]

Men with CP/CPPS are more likely to have genetic alterations that lead to low production of the cytokine, interleukin-10 (IL-10). Differences between CP/CPPS patients and controls also have been reported in the frequency of three alleles near the phosphoglycerate kinase (PGK) gene. The PGK1 gene in the region assessed has been found to be associated with familial prostate cancer, hypospadias (a birth defect leading to an abnormally placed urethra opening in the penis), and androgen insensitivity. Another gene in the same region of the X chromosome encodes the androgen receptor.

Men with CP/CPPS have alterations of both the afferent and efferent autonomic nervous systems. They also have abnormal regulation of the hypothalamic-pituitary-adrenal axis and diurnal cortisol rhythms. Psychological stress also is a common finding in men with CP/CPPS. There are few data on the association of CP/CPPS with erectile dysfunction, though up to one-half of men with CP/CPPS do experience pain with ejaculation.

Adverse prognostic factors for the symptoms of CP/CPPS include stress and psychological function. One study found that greater perceived stress during the 6 months after a health care visit was associated with greater pain intensity and disability at 12 months.[7] Another study correlated worsening symptoms with worsening psychological factors.[8]

Research Priorities and Recommendations

- Develop more data about the natural history of category III prostatitis (i.e., CP/CPPS). This would be very helpful to inform patients and caretakers about expectations and may prevent overtreatment. These studies also may identify specific individuals who will benefit from more intensive early treatment.
- Perform more epidemiologic studies in minority groups. These may identify opportunities for education of patients and physicians about prostatitis and may provide clues about etiology.
- Promote the development of new treatments. To date, no treatments have proved significantly better than placebo for the treatment of CP/CPPS

in randomized trials. This is in part because of a lack of information on the etiology and pathogenesis of this condition. Examination of the above research priorities should provide some starting points for rational, targeted therapy.

- Investigate the association of CP/CPPS with other chronic pelvic pain disorders, such as chronic fatigue syndrome, irritable bowel syndrome, etc.
- Establish criteria to differentiate CP/CPPS from interstitial cystitis (IC)/painful bladder syndrome in epidemiological studies.

Infrastructure Needs of the Community to Allow Progress

- Enhance collaborations with experts from disciplines outside of urology, including genetics, neurology, imaging, pain management, and psychology.
- Investigate the prevalence, incidence, and risk factors for category III prostatitis among different racial and ethnic groups.
- Characterize the natural history, prognostic factors, and clinical course of category III prostatitis. This is especially important for a newly diagnosed disease.
- Foster a better understanding of the risk factors associated with changes in symptoms and progression.
- Standardize definitions for research and clinical trials.
- Explore mechanisms by which an initial infection leads to chronic inflammation despite resolution of the initial infection. There is also an interesting and compelling association between prostate inflammation and subsequent urinary retention, as observed in the NIDDK-sponsored Medical Therapy of Prostate Symptoms (MTOPS) study. This should be further explored.

References:

1. Cheah PY, Liong ML, Yuen KH, et al. Chronic prostatitis: symptom survey with follow-up clinical evaluation. *Urology* 2003;61(1):60–64.

2. McNaughton-Collins M, Joyce GF, Wise M, Pontari MA. Prostatitis. In: Litwin MS, Saigal CS, eds. *Urologic Diseases in America*. U.S. Department of Health and Human Services, National Institutes of Health, National Institute of Diabetes and Digestive and Kidney Diseases. Washington, DC: U.S. Government Printing Office, NIH Publication No. 07-5512: 2007. pp. 9–42.

3. Clemens JQ, Meenan RT, O'Keeffe Rosetti MC, Gao SY, Calhoun EA. Incidence and clinical characteristics of National Institutes of Health type III prostatitis in the community. *Journal of Urology* 2005;174(6):2319–2322.

4. Propert KJ, McNaughton-Collins M, Leiby BE, O'Leary MP, Kusek JW, Litwin MS. A prospective study of symptoms and quality of life in men with chronic prostatitis/chronic pelvic pain syndrome: the National Institutes of Health Chronic Prostatitis Cohort Study. *Journal of Urology* 2006;175(2):619–623.

5. Pontari MA, McNaughton-Collins M, O'Leary MP, et al. A case-control study of risk factors in men with chronic pelvic pain syndrome. *BJU International* 2005;96(4):559–565.

References (continued):

6. Clemens JQ, Meenan RT, O'Keeffe Rosetti MC, Kimes T, Calhoun EA. Prevalence of and risk factors for prostatitis: population-based assessment using physician assigned diagnoses. *Journal of Urology* 2007;178(4 Pt 1):1333-1337.

7. Ullrich PM, Turner JA, Ciol M, Berger R. Stress is associated with subsequent pain and disability among men with nonbacterial prostatitis/pelvic pain. *Annals of Behavioral Medicine* 2005;30(2):112-118.

8. Tripp DA, Nickel JC, Wang Y, et al. Catastrophizing and pain-contingent rest predict patient adjustment in men with chronic prostatitis/chronic pelvic pain syndrome. *The Journal of Pain* 2006;7(10):697-708.

14. Epidemiology of Benign Prostatic Hyperplasia

Over the past several decades, there has been a great deal learned about BPH and its occurrence in the population. Published results have been referenced in several review articles as well as in the *Urologic Diseases in America (UDA)* compendium.[1] In addition, there have been a number of studies on the prevalence on BPH relative to age, race, and ethnicity. A consistent finding is that the prevalence increases with age. By contrast, there is no consistent evidence of a racial or geographic difference in the occurrence of histologic BPH. However, there appears to be some difference in the prevalence of lower urinary tract symptoms (LUTS), but it remains unclear why this difference is seen.

These epidemiologic insights have not been extended to studies of the natural history of BPH/LUTS. However, data are beginning to accumulate on the occurrence of hard outcomes such as treatment or acute urinary retention. Similarly, data are beginning to emerge that better define the progression of LUTS, reduction in flow rates, and increase in prostate volume. There are relatively few longitudinal studies that can provide such insights.

Beyond these very basic observations, there is relatively little consistent information about risk factors for BPH. This is disappointing, as the identification of risk factors is key for moving from a treatment paradigm to disease prevention. Numerous studies have attempted to identify hormonal, lifestyle (e.g., diet and exercise), metabolic, and genetic risk factors. Unfortunately, results from any one study cannot be replicated in others. Moreover, for those few studies that have examined multiple measures of BPH, such as urinary flow rates, prostate size, serum prostate specific antigen (PSA) levels, or others, there have been extremely few risk factors identified as associated with all measures. Thus, there is little from the literature to help develop strategies to prevent the occurrence of BPH.

There are a number of potential factors underlying this lack of progress. First, the lingering effects of a distorted perception that BPH is a normal consequence of aging may have prevented further studies. Similarly, there was a perception that the primary consequence of BPH is a reduction in quality of life (QOL) that men can grow to accept. More recently, however, effective treatments other than surgery have demonstrated that it does not have to be a normal and accepted consequence of aging. In addition, studies have demonstrated that there are important sequelae of BPH that result in significant morbidity.

Perhaps more importantly is that inconsistency in study design may have led to inconsistencies in the risk factors literature. Some of these design factors are related to the selection of the study samples and source populations that are incorrect to address relevant questions. For example, subjects solely recruited from a urology practice will probably not generate insights into risk factors for developing BPH. Similarly, many studies to date have been cross-sectional (i.e., studies at one point in time in a defined population) and, therefore, cannot provide insights into temporal relationships, which is needed for identifying risk factors for BPH development.

Although these design factors have probably contributed to some of the lack of progress, an even greater factor is related to the measurement of BPH itself. Historically, the need for surgical treatment represented the disease phenotype for BPH. More recently, the focus has been on symptom complexes such as those assessed by the International Prostate Symptom Score (IPSS) or American Urological Association Symptom Index (AUASI). This approach is problematic as well because symptoms may be due to multiple etiologies. For example, urinary tract symptoms may be the manifestation of obstruction due to BPH or urethral strictures or resulting from abnormal bladder function. The fact that LUTS represents multiple etiologies is highlighted by the observation that no one pharmaceutical intervention treats all diseases. Thus, progress will require the development of a system to categorize BPH that will take into account the secondary causes of lower urinary tract symptoms, other than BPH.

Research Priorities and Recommendations

- Develop a classification based on new insights into the underlying etiology. This is the number one research priority for epidemiologic studies of BPH. Without this in place, consequent misclassification will likely obscure any potential risk factor associations. To develop this classification system, investigators will need to make use of observations of signs and symptoms of BPH. Importantly, the classification system will need to incorporate etiologic insights from bench and clinical studies. Potential approaches in addition to the traditional studies of mechanical bladder outlet obstruction might include:
1) testing to access hormonal levels, 2) assessment of neurologic and bladder functions, 3) genetic testing for predisposition, and 4) assessments of protein expression. The new system also should incorporate a clarification of the role of comorbid conditions and their influence on disease or alternatively, response to therapy.
- Design future studies to address critical under-lying questions. This includes identifying the appropriate population and sampling schemes. Community samples must be used to determine who develops disease for properly assessing risk factors amenable to prevention. Similarly, it is important to use community-based samples of men with BPH to identify prognostic factors for disease progression. Study samples derived from tertiary care centers or placebo arms of clinical trials should probably not be used to address these questions. Thus, it is necessary to design and assemble cohort

studies to follow men longitudinally to establish temporal and causal relationships and determine who acquires disease versus who has disease. Finally, efforts should ensure that a representative U.S. population is studied.

- Identify risk factors, particularly modifiable risk factors, which may serve as potential targets for intervention, as well as disease prognosis. Although newly identified associations may not always be amenable to intervention or prevention, they may generate hypotheses about etiology.
- Undertake translational studies (Figure 2). The selection of subjects is critical for all studies, whether performed at the population, laboratory, or clinical level. Insights from bench and clinical research could be leveraged to determine how potential risk factors affect the population. Likewise, insights from observed association in population studies may generate new leads for basic science or clinical studies. In fact, it is likely that development of this new paradigm of etiologic-based disease will be evolutionary and progressive and will derive from knowledge gained from basic, clinical, and population-based research.

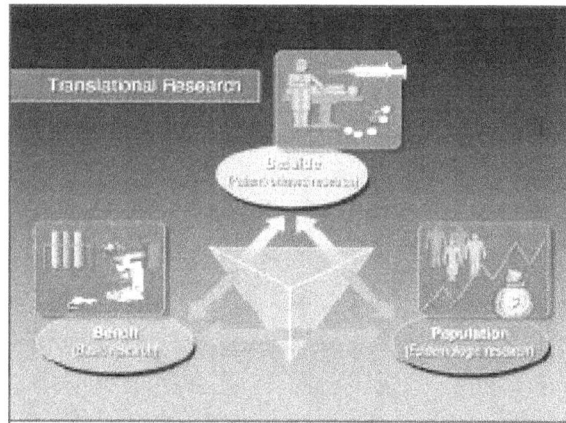

Figure 2. Evolution of care for benign prostatic disease will require tight collaborations and translation of insights between population-based research, basic research, and patient-oriented research/treatment.

Reference:

1. Wei JT, Calhoun EA, Jacobsen SJ. Benign prostatic hyperplasia. In: Litwin MS, Saigal CS, eds. *Urologic Diseases in America*. U.S. Department of Health and Human Services, National Institutes of Health, National Institute of Diabetes and Digestive and Kidney Diseases. Washington, DC: U.S. Government Printing Office, NIH Publication No. 07-5512; 2007. pp. 43-70.

The first point of entry for nearly all men with LUTS is typically the outpatient setting. The UDA project reported an increase in the number of outpatient visits for BPH from 10,116/100,000 in 1994 to 14,473/100,000, while BPH-related visits to emergency rooms declined from 330/100,000 in 1994 to 218/100,000 in 2000.[1] Although the increase in outpatient visits could not be examined based on the available data, one can assume that these visits included clinical evaluations, such as imaging, and prescriptions for medical and surgical interventions. The UDA also reported a dramatic increase in the involvement of primary care physicians in the management of BPH and LUTS (Figure 3), again supporting the contention that our concept of BPH has evolved from an acute surgical condition to a chronic disease.

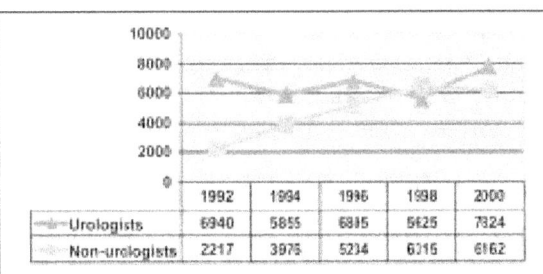

	1992	1994	1996	1998	2000
Urologists	6940	5855	6815	5625	7324
Non-urologists	2217	3976	5234	6215	6162

Figure 3. Increasing role of non-urologists in the care of men with BPH/LUTS (from the NAMCS, 1992, 1994, 1996, 1998, 2000). National trends demonstrates an increasing prevalence of non-urologists (squares) providing care for men with BPH/LUTS while care from urologists (triangles) remain relatively stable during the 1990s. Y axis indicates rates/100,000 male office visits and X axis indicates survey years.[1]

Since the dissemination of the BPH guidelines in 1994, the use of intravenous pyelogram (IVP) and transrectal ultrasound of the prostate in the Medicare population decreased consistently.[2] Computed tomography (CT) scans were uncommonly used in the evaluation of BPH; however, other tests for assessing lower urinary tract function including uroflowmetry and pressure flow studies increased, while the use of cystometrograms decreased modestly. This is substantiated by the 1997 American Urological Association (AUA) Gallup Poll survey of practicing urologists in the United States that reported a decrease in the use of IVP, uroflowmetry, and urodynamic studies.

It is now widely accepted that alpha-blockers and 5-alpha reductase inhibitors are the first-line therapy for symptomatic BPH and LUTS. The AUA Gallup Poll noted that 88 percent of urologists recommended alpha-blockers for men with moderate urinary symptoms and evidence of prostate enlargement of less than 40 cc.[3,4] These findings are supported by data from the NAMCS, which shows that terazosin was the primary pharmacological agent, prescribed in 14 to 15 percent of visits for BPH between 1994 and 1996. With the subsequent introduction of more selective agents, terazosin was replaced by doxazosin and tamsulosin, which together in 2000 constituted 23 percent of the prescriptions written at BPH-related outpatient visits. In contrast, the proportion of outpatient visits in which finasteride was prescribed remained relatively stable (6.5 and 7.3 percent of BPH visits in 1994 and 2000, respectively).

Historically, transurethral resection of the prostate (TURP) was the second most commonly performed operation in the United States for BPH. However, with the introduction of new technology, such as laser vaporization and minimally invasive procedures, practice patterns have evolved significantly since the end of the last decade. Consistent with prior trends, a dramatic decline in hospitalizations for BPH/LUTS was seen throughout the 1990s. Among men over age 65, Medicare data show that outpatient surgery for BPH declined across almost all age, racial/ethnic, and geographic strata of patients. Among those who were hospitalized for BPH surgery, lengths of stay were shorter, consistent with trends following widespread adoption of prospective payment and managed care systems. With the use of laser procedures instead of TURP, it is likely that these trends are even pronounced today.

In the 1990s, minimally invasive surgical therapies (MIST) were introduced. These include laser ablation, transurethral needle ablation (TUNA), transurethral microwave therapy (TUMT), high-energy focused ultrasound, and hot-water thermotherapy. The 1997 AUA Gallup Poll of practicing urologists indicated that while 95 percent had performed TURP in the prior year, 26 percent had performed a laser prostatectomy. Only 3 percent had performed TUNA or TUMT. According to data from the Health Cost and Utilization Project, of the MIST procedures performed in the inpatient setting, only TUNA and TUMT increased by the end of the decade while the use of laser prostatectomy has declined. Simultaneously, BPH procedures in an ambulatory surgery setting increased substantially toward the end of the decade.

Research Priorities and Recommendations

* Conduct reviews of administrative data (e.g., the UDA program) to aid the monitoring of practice patterns and quality of care. Such programs need to be developed consistently with current NIH efforts.
* Develop large prospective cohort studies of contemporary practice patterns because such administrative data are often limited. These should be nationally representative when possible and powered to permit analyses of racial/ethnic groups and various socioeconomic strata.
* Promote urologic health services researchers interested in examining clinical epidemiology, economics, and quality of care. Support of career

development/training and other programs that promote this among urology residents should be fostered. Centers of excellence for training urologic health services researchers should be established for long-term viability of these efforts.
* Quality of care indicators for BPH should be evaluated, disseminated, and then tracked over time. This is especially important in light of the persistent variation in the management of BPH. Also, this priority is particularly relevant given the rise in primary care provider involvement.
* Examine the appropriateness of medical management. For example, how often are men treated with medical management that is ineffective, yet patients are not instructed to discontinue? Use of combination therapy has been shown to be effective yet is largely limited to a small percentage of men followed by urologists.

References:

1. Wei JT, Calhoun E, Jacobsen SJ. Urologic diseases in America project: benign prostatic hyperplasia. *Journal of Urology* 2005;173(4):1256–1261.

2. McConnell JD, Barry MJ, Bruskewitz, R.C. et al. *Benign Prostatic Hyperplasia: Diagnosis and Treatment. Clinical Practice Guideline No. 8.* AHCPR Pub. No. 94-0582. Rockville, MD: Agency for Health Care Policy and Research, Public Health Service, U.S. Department of Health and Human Services; 1994.

3. Gee WF, Holtgrewe HL, Blute ML, et al. 1997 American Urological Association Gallup survey: changes in diagnosis and management of prostate cancer and benign prostatic hyperplasia, and other practice trends from 1994 to 1997. *Journal of Urology* 1998;160(5):1804–1807.

4. Gee WF, Holtgrewe HL, Albertsen PC, et al. Practice trends in the diagnosis and management of benign prostatic hyperplasia in the United States. *Journal of Urology* 1995;154(1):205–206.

16. Practice Patterns for Prostatitis

Few systematic investigations have been performed to assess practice patterns for the management of men with category III prostatitis (i.e., chronic prostatitis/chronic pelvic pain syndrome, CP/CPPS). The studies that have been performed to date are summarized below.

As part of the CPCRN cohort study, patients with CP/CPPS were queried about previous treatments. Results are provided in Table 1.[1]

One study surveyed Canadian urologists to assess practice patterns for CP/CPPS, epidididymitis, and IC.[2] Results are summarized in Table 2.

Another study surveyed 290 primary care physicians about practice patterns related to CP/CPPS.[3] Approximately one-half (48 percent) of physicians were "not at all" familiar with the NIH classification

of prostatitis, and 33 percent reported "never" having seen such a patient. Fully 65 percent of respondents correctly identified the hallmark symptom of CP/CPPS (i.e., pelvic pain). Regarding etiology, 71 percent correctly indicated that CP/CPPS was non-infectious, 37 percent incorrectly reported that it was caused by a sexually transmitted disease, and 35 percent incorrectly indicated that it was caused by a psychiatric illness. Male physicians and physicians who see a higher percent of male patients answered more of these questions correctly. Management strategies are presented in Table 3.

A randomized controlled trial from the CPCRN showed that antibiotics and alpha-blockers are not effective in men previously treated with these agents.[4] There are no data to support the efficacy of long treatment courses, while the risk of side effects increases with prolonged administration.

Table 1. Prevalence of previous procedures and treatments for CPPS reported at baseline screening in 488 CPC study participants.

	No. (Percent)
Previous procedures:	
Cystoscopy	259 (53.73)
Other	164 (34.82)
Bladder hydrodistention	44 (9.69)
Urethral dilation	29 (6)
Chronic pelvic pain syndrome treatment before or at screening:	
Antibiotics or antimicrobials	464 (95.08)
Anti-inflammatory medicine	319 (66.46)
Plant extracts or herbs	267 (54.71)
Zinc	230 (47.62)
α-Blockers	202 (42.44)
Prostate massage	196 (38.19)
Special diet or nutritional supplements	169 (34.7)
Antidepressants	102 (21.16)
Anti-anxiety medications	99 (19.5)
5α-reductase inhibitors	96 (19.53)
Other	95 (17.63)
Stress reduction techniques	79 (16.05)
Narcotics	74 (15.23)
Urinary tract analgesics	70 (14.68)
Anticholinergics or antispasmodics	67 (14.53)
Acupuncture or acupressure	65 (13.32)
Steroids	50 (10.31)
Electrical stimulation	33 (6.8)
Biofeedback	27 (5.57)
Allopurinol	19 (3.78)
Anticonvulsants	16 (3.35)

Research Priorities and Recommendations

* Educate primary care physicians on proper diagnosis. Many men with CP/CPPS would indicate that an early, accurate diagnosis for their symptoms is an unmet need. The psychological benefit is enormous for many, even though we currently lack effective treatments.
* Identification of areas of poor quality care. This may help to reduce unnecessary costs, as well as treatment side effects. Two potential areas of overtreatment include the long-term (> 6 weeks) use of antimicrobials for CP/CPPS and the use of alpha-blockers or antimicrobials in men who have previously failed this treatment.
* Examine primary care physician knowledge and practice patterns regarding CP/CPPS. Many men with CP/CPPS initially present to a primary care physician. Better education of physicians may facilitate an earlier diagnosis and may improve outcomes in men with CP/CPPS.
* Educate primary care physicians on the basic principles that differentiate the three major prostate diseases (i.e., prostate cancer, BPH, and prostatitis).
* Perform a systematic assessment of urology practice patterns regarding CP/CPPS. This may identify patterns of overtreatment that could be the targets of cost reduction strategies.

Table 2. Most common investigations and treatments previously performed, used, prescribed, or planned.

	Prostatitis (percent in parentheses)	Interstitial Cystitis (percent in parentheses)	Epididymitis (percent in parentheses)
Investigations	Urinalysis (67)	Urinalysis (64)	Urinalysis (65)
	Urine cultures (64)	Urine cultures (57)	Urine cultures (65)
	Cystoscopy (49)	Cystoscopy (48)	Cystoscopy (47)
	Ultrasound (26)	Ultrasound (24)	Ultrasound (25)
	Urodynamics (19)	Urodynamics (19)	Urodynamics (23)
Treatments	Antibiotics (74)	Antibiotics (73 percent)	Antibiotics (75)
	α-blockers (29)	Anti-inflammatories (24)	Anti-inflammatories (40)
	Anti-inflammatories (25)	Anticholinergics (22)	Anticholinergics (32)
	Pentosan polysulfate (20 percent)	Pentosan polysulfate (19)	Pentosan polysulfate (23)
	Anti-anxiolytics (20 percent)	Intravesical treatment (13)	Anti-anxiolytics (21)

Table 3. Management/Treatment Strategies.

Management/Treatment	Almost Always (percent)	More than ½ of the Time (percent)	About ½ of the Time (percent)	Less than ½ of the Time (percent)	Rarely (percent)	Never (percent)
Refer to specialist	9.2	16.1	16.1	19.5	29.9	9.2
Test for *Neisseria gonorrhoeae* and *Chlamydia*	70.9	15.4	4.9	6.0	1.6	1.1
Post-void residual	5.6	6.7	6.1	17.3	33.5	30.7
Serum creatinine	40.0	18.9	9.4	8.3	16.1	7.2
CT scan of abdomen and pelvis	3.9	6.1	9.5	10.6	48.0	21.8
Pre- and post-prostate massage urine cultures	12.8	10.6	7.3	8.9	26.8	33.5
Serum PSA	21.5	19.2	9.0	9.0	20.9	20.3
Prostate ultrasound	2.8	5.6	10.2	14.1	33.9	33.3
Antibiotics	37.2	35.0	11.1	7.2	4.4	5.0
α-blockers	2.3	19.2	19.2	13.6	21.5	24.3
5-α reductase inhibitors	0.6	0.6	6.2	6.2	19.8	66.7
Non-steroidal anti-inflammatory drugs	17.4	29.2	15.2	9.6	15.2	13.5
Antidepressants	0.6	2.2	8.4	14.0	32.4	42.5
Anticholinergics	0.6	3.9	5.0	15.1	34.6	40.9
Complementary/alternative therapies	1.7	1.7	2.8	10.1	25.8	57.9

References:

1. Schaeffer AJ, Landis JR, Knauss JS, et al. Demographic and clinical characteristics of men with chronic prostatitis: the National Institutes of Health Chronic Prostatitis Cohort Study. *Journal of Urology* 2002;168(2):593–598.

2. Nickel JC, Teichman JM, Gregoire M, Clark J, Downey J. Prevalence, diagnosis, characterization, and treatment of prostatitis, interstitial cystitis, and epididymitis in outpatient urological practice: the Canadian PIE Study. *Urology* 2005;66(5):935–940.

3. Clemens JQ, Calhoun EA, Litwin MS, Collins MM. Primary care physician practice patterns in the management of chronic prostatitis/chronic pelvic pain syndrome. *Journal of Urology* 2007;177(4 Suppl):30–31.

4. Alexander RB, Propert KJ, Schaeffer AJ, et al. Ciprofloxacin or tamsulosin in men with chronic prostatitis/chronic pelvic pain syndrome: a randomized, double-blind trial. *Annals of Internal Medicine* 2004;141(8):581–589.

17. Quality of Care for Benign Prostatic Hyperplasia and Prostatitis

As medical costs have risen, there is a growing demand for more efficient cost-conscious health care without compromising quality.[1,2] The medical profession has responded by initiating research to document appropriateness of medical treatment and better define quality of care.[2] One study proposed measuring available medical resources, technical aspects of care, and outcomes as an evaluation of patients' health status. This paradigm has become the basis for research in health care quality assessment.[3]

Geographic variation in use of health care services has been demonstrated in a variety of medical conditions, prompting concern over the underlying reasons for clinical decisions. The most widely disparate treatment rates have been observed in situations where physicians disagree on the utility of competing approaches.[4] One of the most prominently cited examples of regional variation is the rate of TURP. One study provided information about six northeastern states and found that rates for some surgeries, including TURP, varied by two-to-six-fold.[4] The predominant factor appeared to be the physician's assessment of treatment utility.

Quality of Care for BPH

Data from the UDA project reveal that national spending related to BPH was $1.1 billion in 2000. BPH-related office visits were 14,473 per 100,000 males in the same year.[5] Therefore, a large portion of any primary care physician's or urologist's practice consists of BPH management. Practice variations in diagnosis and treatment continue to exist in spite of the widespread access to information via the internet and the evidence-based medicine movement. Surgical and medical therapies continue to vary at the county, state, and national level.[6] To minimize practice variation, physicians are encouraged to use tools such as the Cochrane Library, American College of Physicians Journal Club, or national guidelines to inform their treatment decision making. Unfortunately, if only low level evidence exists for a given topic, these tools will be of minimum benefit (e.g., the Cochrane library has only one systematic review on BPH surgical therapy). Although BPH guidelines are available, the methodology and recommendations are not uniform.[7] Perhaps this disparity accounts for the finding that two-thirds of primary care physicians were not in accordance with the Agency for Healthcare Policy and Research BPH guidelines.[8] Guidelines themselves vary in their usability as well.

The most recent focus for improving care is accountability from hospitals and physicians. Institutions and physicians have been hesitant to initiate voluntary quality reporting because of concerns as to how quality is measured. The Hospital Quality Initiative and the Physician Voluntary Reporting Program have been developed as incentives to change behavior. The Centers for Medicare and Medicaid are linking reimbursement to high-quality care. As these initiatives expand, it would benefit the urology community to develop quality indicators that are feasible, reasonable, and not prohibitively expensive. Twelve quality indicators for BPH have been developed specifically for vulnerable elders and are in press in the *Journal of the American Geriatric Society*.[9]

Quality of Care for Prostatitis

A major quality of care issue for CP/CPPS is the overuse of antibiotics. CP/CPPS pelvic pain and voiding symptoms are similar to those that occur with a true bacterial infection. Therefore, it is not surprising that one of the most common theories of etiology is that of an occult infection. However, only 5 to 10 percent of cases of CP/CPPS are caused by active infection. There are data to suggest that infection, especially sexually transmitted disease, may be a risk

factor for the development of CP/CPPS[10], but there is not a significant number of men with CP/CPPS in which an ongoing infection can be diagnosed.[11] In the CPCRN study, in response to questions on previous or concurrent treatments for the chronic pelvic pain syndrome, 95 percent of subjects reported antibiotics or antimicrobial use.[12] According to the NAMCS database in 1992 to 2000, the most common medications associated with any visits for prostatitis were quinolones (an annualized rate of 319/100,000), followed by sulfa medications (an annualized rate of 287/100,000) and then BPH medications (an annualized rate of 91/100,000). When visits for infectious prostatitis were removed from the data, the rates of prescribing quinolones and sulfa medications remained essentially the same.[13] Common practice is to offer a course of antibiotics, even in patients who may not have a documented infection. However, repeated courses of antibiotics for symptoms of pelvic pain are likely inappropriate, given the lack of data on the efficacy of a repeat course in this situation, the expense, and certainly the risk of adverse effects.

Research Priorities and Recommendations

- Support a year of research related to benign prostatic disease as one way to foster future academic pursuits of young urologists. Economic and other constraints have contributed to a loss of the traditional research year in many urology training programs. Existing NIH workshops focusing on clinical research career development in urology should be continued to maintain enthusiasm among young faculty attempting to succeed as independent researchers. Networking and collaboration beyond the AUA alone is crucial.
- Encourage active research cooperatives such as the Urinary Incontinence Treatment Network (or develop new cooperatives similar to the MTOPS) to sponsor the randomized controlled trials needed to answer efficacy questions.
- Generate quality indicators that may be used both inside and outside the United States. This would increase the generalizability of the indicators and potentially strengthen their appeal.
- Develop large, randomized controlled trials and nationally representative, observational studies to address efficacy issues among BPH therapies, but particularly minimally invasive modalities. There is a current paucity of high-level evidence delineating the appropriate surgical treatment for different subpopulations of men with BPH symptoms.

48

These studies should include sufficient granularity for patient-centered outcomes, etiologies, and risk factors so that adjustment for confounding is possible.

- Develop studies that help to realign efficacy with reimbursement. These would help control long-term costs.
- Address the differences in BPH management guidelines among different organizations, particularly between Americans and their European counterparts.
- Improve the objective, validated longitudinal evaluation of urinary frequency, urgency, urinary incontinence, nocturia, decreased force of stream, feeling of incomplete bladder emptying, or post void dribbling (i.e., LUTS). The CPSI is currently underused. Non-academic family practitioners and urologists should be encouraged to use these standardized, validated objective assessment tools.
- Estimate the degree of antibiotic overuse for CP/CPPS.
- Investigate the incidence of treatable lesions (such as bladder carcinoma *in situ*, urethral stricture, or undiagnosed neurologic lesions) in men initially diagnosed with CP/CPPS.

References:

1. Brook RH, Lohr K, Chassin M, Kosecoff J, Fink A, Solomon D. Geographic variations in the use of services: do they have any clinical significance? *Health Affairs (Project Hope)* 1984;3(2):63–73.

2. Hay J, Leahy MJ. Physician-induced demand: an empirical analysis of the consumer information gap. *Journal of Health Economics* 1982;1(3):231–244.

3. Donabedian A. Quality assurance. Structure, process and outcome. *Nursing Standard* 1992;7(11 Suppl QA):4–5.

4. Wennberg J, Gittelsohn A. Variations in medical care among small areas. *Scientific American* 1982;246(4):120–134.

5. Wei JT, Calhoun E, Jacobsen SJ. Urologic diseases in America project: benign prostatic hyperplasia. *Journal of Urology* 2005;173(4):1256–1261.

6. Sung JC, Curtis LH, Schulman KA, Albala DM. Geographic variations in the use of medical and surgical therapies for benign prostatic hyperplasia. *Journal of Urology* 2006;175(3 Pt 1):1023–1027.

7. Irani J, Brown CT, van der MJ, Emberton M. A review of guidelines on benign prostatic hyperplasia and lower urinary tract symptoms: are all guidelines the same? *BJU International* 2003;92(9):937–942.

8. Collins MM, Barry MJ, Bin L, Roberts RG, Oesterling JE, Fowler FJ. Diagnosis and treatment of benign prostatic hyperplasia. Practice patterns of primary care physicians. *Journal of General Internal Medicine* 1997;12(4):224–229.

9. Saigal CS. Quality indicators for benign prostatic hyperplasia in vulnerable elders. *Journal of the American Geriatrics Society* 2007;55 Suppl 2:S253–S257.

10. Pontari MA, McNaughton-Collins M, O'Leary MP, et al. A case-control study of risk factors in men with chronic pelvic pain syndrome. *BJU International* 2005;96(4):559–565.

11. Weidner W, Schiefer HG, Krauss H, Jantos C, Friedrich HJ, Altmannsberger M. Chronic prostatitis: a thorough search for etiologically involved microorganisms in 1,461 patients. *Infection* 1991;19(Suppl 3):S119–S125.

12. Schaeffer AJ, Landis JR, Knauss JS, et al. Demographic and clinical characteristics of men with chronic prostatitis: the National Institutes of Health Chronic Prostatitis Cohort Study. *Journal of Urology* 2002;168(2):593–598.

13. Pontari MA, Joyce GF, Wise M, McNaughton-Collins M. Prostatitis. *Journal of Urology* 2007;177(6):2050–2057.

18. Diffusion of New Technology for Benign Prostatic Hyperplasia and Prostatitis

Observational studies of practice patterns in the U.S. population provide most of what is currently known about the diffusion of novel therapies for benign prostate disease. These studies include Gallup polls of practicing urologists[1] and observational analyses of large datasets (e.g., Medicare, the NAMCS, and the Healthcare Cost and Utilization Project).[2] Although these analyses provide descriptions of trends in the use of new treatments, they provide limited insight on different variables that shape these trends.

Thus, while we know something about the *outcomes* of technology diffusion, we know much less about the *process* of diffusion (i.e., how or why diffusion of particular therapies occurs). For example, over the last decade medical therapies for BPH have gained while surgical therapies declined in incidence.[3] However, our understanding of the forces that shaped this trend remains limited, as does our ability to predict how this trend will affect long-term patient outcomes.

49

Indeed, a prominent shortcoming in current clinical research for benign prostate disease is the dearth of attention paid to assessing long-term clinical efficacy when a new and unproven therapy—particularly a novel technology—diffuses rapidly into clinical practice. A potential pitfall in this regard is the dispersion of an unproven therapy that outpaces the collection and analysis of objective outcomes data.

Greater understanding of the variables that drive, impede, or otherwise influence the diffusion of a novel therapy after it is introduced into urological practice—variables that include provider characteristics, patient characteristics, marketing, the media, the Internet, and sociologic pressures—would potentially optimize the efficient delivery of the latest, most effective, most cost-efficient health care for BPH and prostatitis (Figure 4).[3]

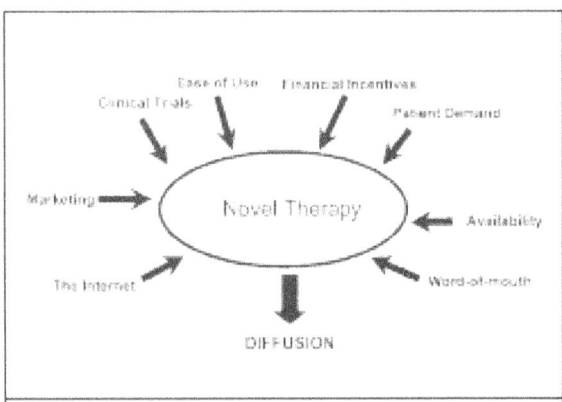

Figure 4 Variables that potentially influence the diffusion of a new therapy into clinical practice.

Research Priorities and Recommendations

- Assess how new therapies diffuse through populations. This will require increased partnership with other academic disciplines, including economics, sociology, psychology, and communications. These partnerships should explore:
  - How trends in treatment develop and spread through populations, both at the provider and patient levels.
  - How clinical practice intersects with industry and the media in this regard.
- Develop research opportunities to explore:
  - The intersection of urological practice with the social sciences—particularly economics, sociology, and communications.

- Novel methods of modeling and predicting long-term outcomes resulting from current treatment preferences and patterns.
- Refine and expand observational studies of current practice patterns. This should incorporate:
  - Increased reliance on evidence-based medicine and objective outcomes data.
  - Cost/benefit analyses for use of new technology—particularly for those therapies with lucrative economic benefits for manufacturers and health care providers.
  - A public access database, mandatory for all devices, to address the lack of sufficient data on complications.
  - Use of health maintenance organization (HMO) datasets.
  - Practice trend analyses by region, practitioner, patient demographics, types of health care plan, availability of new technologies, and other variables.
  - Promotion of validated patient safety indicators and other validated measures for assessing complications and other issues related to patient safety.[4]
  - Patient surveys and preference analyses.
- Develop novel models, instruments, and metrics for studying variables that potentially influence the diffusion of novel treatments. Studies should address:
  - Economic trends, incentives (provider and patient), costs, and marketing of new therapies by industry.
  - Availability of technology, provider education/background, and complexity of additional training required for using a new device.
  - The process by which providers are certified to use new devices: the organizations/entities that oversee or maintain certification, the training curriculum, number of cases required to be certified, need for a proctor, and whether a professional organization (i.e., the AUA) or other third party is involved.
  - Patient preferences and the decision-making process (e.g., how patients chose a particular treatment).
  - The influence of patient preference in driving new technologies.
  - The sociologic dynamics by which knowledge of a novel therapy spreads through patient populations and popular culture (e.g., press releases, advertising, the Internet, tipping points, and word-of-mouth).

- Promote multidisciplinary collaborations to study the diffusion of new technology so that it does not outpace rigorously obtained outcomes, efficacy, and safety data.

- Measure long-term clinical efficacy (i.e., durability of effect) using the above approaches.

References:

1. Gee WF, Holtgrewe HL, Blute ML, et al. 1997 American Urological Association Gallup Survey: changes in diagnosis and management of prostate cancer and benign prostatic hyperplasia, and other practice trends from 1994 to 1997. *Journal of Urology* 1998;160(5):1804–1807.

2. Wei JT, Calhoun E, Jacobsen SJ. Urologic diseases in America project: benign prostatic hyperplasia. *Journal of Urology* 2005;173(4):1256–1261.

3. Pontari MA, Joyce GF, Wise M, McNaughton-Collins M. Prostatitis. *Journal of Urology* 2007;177(6):2050–2057.

4. Miller MR, Elixhauser A, Zhan C, Meyer GS. Patient safety indicators: using administrative data to identify potential patient safety concerns. *Health Services Research* 2001;36(6 Pt 2):110–132.

19. Quality of Life for Benign Prostatic Hyperplasia and Prostatitis

Quality of Life in BPH

Despite the public health and economic importance of BPH, relatively little work has been done to understand factors that cause a man to seek medical attention for his urinary symptoms. The decision to seek care is complex and involves not only the recognition of symptoms, but also the impact of symptoms, decisions about whether symptoms are indicative of disease, are treatable, and whether treatment benefits outweigh risks. Previous studies have suggested that presence of symptoms alone is not enough to trigger health care seeking behavior.[1,2,3] For urinary dysfunction, symptoms in fact, actually explain only a small portion of variance in health care-seeking behavior. Age, perceived bother, and embarrassment about urinary function are stronger predictors of whether a patient will seek treatment. These data suggest that there are strong psychosocial components to the decision to seek care for urinary symptoms beyond just the occurrence of urinary symptoms.

Although the tools for direct symptom measurement are widely used, higher order health measurement questions can be used to directly inquire about the impact, importance, bother, or QOL issues associated with symptoms from the patient's perspective. These may ultimately be more useful in determining treatment strategies and health care utilization. Studies examining health-related QOL instruments suggest that men with urologic dysfunction report a wide range of factors that impact QOL (e.g., reductions in psychologic well-being, restrictions in daily activities and social relationships, increased levels of physical symptoms, and a decrease in general health perceptions). Furthermore, there is considerable variation in how urinary symptoms are perceived and affect daily life. Irritative symptoms (e.g., urgency, frequency, nocturia, and incontinence), because of their greater bother, tend to cause the most impairment, whereas symptoms related to obstructions in the lower urinary tract (e.g., terminal dribbling and hesitancy) tend to have the least effect on QOL. Finally, urinary symptoms tend to be more strongly associated with overall health status and QOL measures than with objective measures of condition severity, such as anatomic and urodynamic parameters.

These findings indicate the usefulness of collecting QOL information for the evaluation and management of benign prostate disease. Multiple types of measures are needed in the assessment of patients for informed decision-making and the evaluation of treatment outcomes. Although clinicians have tended to rely more on objective, clinical measures in assessing condition severity and making treatment decisions, the most important indicators appear to be the impact of symptoms on QOL and treatment preferences. This would represent a change in treatment criteria, particularly for BPH.

QOL for Prostatitis

The issue of QOL for prostatitis has been increasingly studied in the last 10 years. The CPCRN study used the SF-12 questionnaire as a measure of QOL. In the CPCRN, CP/CPPS patients' Mental Component Scores were lower than those observed in the most severe subgroups of patients with congestive heart failure and diabetes mellitus.[4] History of psychiatric disease and younger age were strongly associated with worse scores. Physical domain scores were worse than those among the general U.S. male population, and specifically a history of rheumatologic disease was associated with worse physical QOL scores. The NIH-CPSI includes a QOL subscale, in addition to questions about pain and urinary symptoms. Predictors of poor QOL include urinary symptoms, depression as measured by a separate depression index, and pain intensity.[5] Prostatitis also leads men to seek medical treatment. In the recent UDA study, combined physician outpatient and hospital outpatient visits revealed an age-adjusted, annualized visit rate for prostatitis of 1,798/100,000 population.[6] Whereas in men with BPH, it is predominantly LUTS that drives visitation to a physician; in men with CP/CPPS, it could be LUTS and/or pelvic pain. The contribution of LUTS versus the pain component to seeking medical attention has not been addressed in men with CP/CPPS.

Research Priorities and Recommendations

- Improve dissemination of research findings, user-friendly QOL instruments, and physician education programs for using better QOL measures in clinical practice.
- Establish Health Services Research Training Programs for urology residents. This would focus attention on this important area of research and would provide the necessary theoretical and methodological training and mentoring for trainees to develop successful clinical research careers. These training programs should include training in epidemiology, quality of care, and QOL issues.
- Develop research protocols related to QOL for prostate disorders.
- Develop and evaluate further generic and condition-specific measures of lower urinary tract dysfunctions. Published reports of instruments

should provide information about the psychometric properties of the measures, as well as their performance in subgroups of the population (e.g., gender, ethnicity, educational levels, age groups, and homebound/nursing home versus community dwelling).

- Promote additional epidemiologic and observational research concerning lower urinary tract dysfunction. These could be strengthened by including QOL measures. It is important to delineate more clearly the factors that determine the extent to which men are bothered by urinary/pain symptoms and to determine how these affect QOL. The relationship of comorbidities to urologic dysfunction and QOL also needs to be examined. In addition, population-based studies of lower urinary tract dysfunction may help us better understand the treatment-seeking behavior of patients with these conditions, because a majority of older adults do not seek treatment for these problems.
- Incorporate QOL instruments in the assessment of treatment effectiveness. Selection of appropriate instruments should be based on the goals of the investigations, the domains of interest, and the psychometric properties of the measures (i.e., reliability, validity, and sensitivity to changes in clinical status). This would necessitate QOL assessment before the initiation of treatment and at periodic intervals during the course of therapy. Not only should the QOL questionnaires evaluate the domains of interest, but also they must be sufficiently sensitive to detect changes in health status as a result of treatment. Monitoring QOL for a longer period would be important in those conditions for which ongoing treatment is necessary. Such questionnaires can be easily incorporated in clinical practice by having the patient complete a self-administered questionnaire during an office visit.

References:

1. Girman CJ, Jacobsen SJ, Tsukamoto T, et al. Health-related quality of life associated with lower urinary tract symptoms in four countries. *Urology* 1998;51(3):428–436.

2. Roberts RO, Rhodes T, Panser LA, et al. Natural history of prostatism: worry and embarrassment from urinary symptoms and health care-seeking behavior. *Urology* 1994;43(5):621–628.

3. Girman CJ, Jacobsen SJ, Rhodes T, Guess HA, Roberts RO, Lieber MM. Association of health-related quality of life and benign prostatic enlargement. *European Urology* 1999;35(4):277–284.

4. McNaughton CM, Pontari MA, O'Leary MP, et al. Quality of life is impaired in men with chronic prostatitis: the Chronic Prostatitis Collaborative Research Network. *Journal of General Internal Medicine* 2001;16(10):656–662.

5. Tripp DA, Curtis NJ, Landis JR, Wang YL, Knauss JS. Predictors of quality of life and pain in chronic prostatitis/chronic pelvic pain syndrome: findings from the National Institutes of Health Chronic Prostatitis Cohort Study. *BJU International* 2004;94(9):1279–1282.

6. Pontari MA, Joyce GF, Wise M, McNaughton-Collins M. Prostatitis. *Journal of Urology* 2007;177(6):2050–2057.

Direct versus Indirect Costs

Direct costs refer to costs associated with office visits, inpatient hospitalizations, ambulatory surgery, emergency department visits, and prescription medications. Sources of direct costs include room and board, laboratory, pharmacy, radiographic studies, physician professional fees, and operating department costs. Indirect costs include work absenteeism, decreased productivity, and economic disruption in other roles (e.g., needing helpers to complete regular tasks).

Cost of BPH Care

BPH, and its associated clinical manifestation of LUTS, is listed among the most common medical conditions of aging men. Estimates of national expenditures for BPH care vary from $2 to $4 billion per year over the past decade and a half.[1,2,3] In the early 1990s, one researcher estimated that $4 billion was spent annually on BPH treatment with approximately $575 million paid in professional fees.[3] Based on claims data, another article calculated the direct cost of BPH care to the private sector (i.e., privately insured men age 45–64 years) at $3.4 billion dollars in 1999.[4] However, the UDA project reported the direct cost of medical services excluding outpatient pharmaceuticals as a modest $1.1 billion for 2000.[5] Medicare costs for BPH through the 1990s have decreased by 31 percent ($1.1 billion in 1992 to $776 million in 1998). As Medicare has not covered prescription drugs until 2006, these numbers reflect a shift in the burden of expenditures from the government to patients. The decline in Medicare spending is mainly attributable to a significant reduction in inpatient expenditures. In nominal dollars, total hospital spending for BPH among Medicare beneficiaries decreased by 58 percent from $743 million in 1992 to $315 million in 1998.[5]

The decline in inpatient spending for BPH mirrors other components of BPH care. From 1996–1998, average annual spending on BPH pharmaceuticals was $194 million. By 2002, more than $600 million was spent on finasteride and tamsulosin alone, representing an increase of more than 200 percent.[5,6] Physician office expenditures for BPH rose 12.4 percent, from $291.2 million in 1992 to $327.5 million in 1998. Similarly, ambulatory surgery expenditures for BPH increased by 37 percent, from $73.4 million in 1992 to $100.3 in 1998. Emergency department costs

for BPH also grew 25 percent from $15.5 million in 1992 to $19.8 million in 1998.[7] The incremental cost per patient per year associated with a BPH diagnosis was $1,536 in 1999.[4] More recently, an article published in the *American Journal of Managed Care* conducted a descriptive, retrospective study of health care utilization costs during the first year of BPH using PharMetrics, a patient-centric database from 1999–2002 and 2003 cost estimates.[8] This database consisted of 61 U.S. health plans and focused on newly diagnosed BPH patients. Costs for medications, physician visits, ER visits, screening and monitoring tests, surgery, and complications were considered. The total national direct cost estimate was $3 billion per year.

The cost effectiveness and cost utility of finasteride, doxazosin, and combination therapy for moderate to severe BPH also has been evaluated.[9] Using a semi-Markov decision analytic model and considering rates for acute urinary retentions (AUR), BPH-related surgeries, and deaths, researchers assigned quality adjusted life years (QALYs) and cost consequence (e.g., cost per AUR or TURP avoided) to determine the cost utilities of single and combination therapy (i.e., cost per QALY gained). The incremental cost per AUR & TURP averted (finasteride relative to doxazosin) was $83,089 and $14,047, respectively. The incremental cost per AUR & TURP averted was $88,400 and $22,478, respectively. Their cost-utility analysis (relative to doxazosin) suggested that finasteride may have less benefit at higher cost, while combination treatment may have greater benefit (cost per QALY gained $34,085) at higher cost.

One study modeled the long-term cost-effectiveness of BPH treatment, watchful waiting, medical therapy (i.e., alpha-blockers, 5-alpha-reductase inhibitors, or combination), and surgery (i.e., TUMT or TURP) using a Markov decision analysis.[10] They found that the use of alpha-blockers for moderate symptoms and TURP for severe symptoms are preferred strategies. They also suggested that TUMT may be useful in the short term for moderate symptoms but not cost-effective over the long term.

The economic burden of BPH also may be characterized by its indirect costs in terms of absenteeism, work limitations, and premature mortality. Privately insured men 45 to 64 years old with a diagnosis of

BPH missed an average of 7.3 hours of work per year due to the condition with more than 10 percent reporting some work loss or temporary disability.[4] Outpatient visits accounted for the majority of lost work time, with an average of 4.7 hours of work lost per visit. Approximately 2.2 million men age 45 to 64 years in the work force who receive treatment for BPH led to 2 million lost work days and an indirect cost of BPH care borne by the private sector alone estimated at $500 million per year.[4]

Cost of Prostatitis Care

In the United States, an estimated $84 million was spent on treating prostatitis in 2000, according to inpatient and outpatient claims of patients with a primary diagnosis of prostatitis. This estimate consists of $35 million for inpatient services, $24 million for ambulatory surgery, $16 million for emergency department visits, and $4 million for hospital outpatient visits. Treatment costs of prostatitis have increased over time. Between 1994 and 2002, mean costs increased for emergency department visits, physician outpatient visits, and inpatient hospitalization. In 2002, the average annual expenditure for privately insured individuals aged 18 to 64 years with a medical claim corresponding to a diagnosis of prostatitis was $5,464 ($4,038 for medical care and $1,426 for prescription drugs) and $3,704 for insured individuals without a medical claim relating to prostatitis. The difference in expenditure ($1,759) is likely accounted for by costs directly or indirectly related to prostatitis.[11]

One study used administrative data from the Kaiser Permanente Northwest HMO to compare costs incurred by 5,241 men with prostatitis with costs incurred by a control group matched for age.[12] Prostatitis was defined based on a diagnosis of "chronic prostatitis" or "prostatitis not otherwise specified." Prescription costs, prescription fills, outpatient and inpatient costs, and inpatient stays were all greater for patients with prostatitis than for controls. The mean annual cost for patients with prostatitis was $4,387, and the mean annual total cost for the control population was $2,689. The difference in total cost was due primarily to outpatient and pharmacy expenses.

Another researcher reported similar findings in a study using Group Health Cooperative HMO data in Washington State.[13] Mean costs for 270 men with a new diagnosis of prostatitis were significantly greater than costs for age-matched controls in both the year preceding ($2,134 versus $1,469) and the year subsequent to the diagnosis ($2,410 versus $1,728). However, when costs specific to prostatitis (e.g., medications and typical diagnostic tests such as urinalysis and cystoscopy) were calculated, these were only a small proportion of the total observed costs. These findings suggest that seeking care for prostatitis is part of a broader pattern of health care use for multiple medical problems. The 10 percent of patients with prostatitis with the greatest total costs accounted for about one-half of all costs.

Costs Assessments for CP/CPPS from the CPC Study

The CPCRN is an ongoing, multicenter project funded by the NIH to study category III prostatitis (i.e., CP/CPPS). An initial CPCRN project was the establishment of the Chronic Prostatitis Cohort (CPC), which consisted of 488 men with CP/CPPS who were followed longitudinally. The direct and indirect costs associated with CP/CPPS were examined in a subset of 167 of these men.[14] Fully 82 percent of these men had accrued some costs over the 3-month period prior to their enrollment in the cohort. The average man had undergone six procedures, had five physician visits, and taken two and a half prescriptions for his condition over the 3-month period. Of the men enrolled, 80 percent incurred direct costs and 26 percent had indirect costs. Procedures and tests (mean of $761) were the largest component of directs costs, followed by health care visits (mean of $325) and medication (mean of $282). Their average total costs (direct plus indirect) related to CP/CPPS for the 3-month period prior to enrollment in the study was $1,099 per person, with a projected annual total cost (direct and indirect) of $4,397 per person. This cost is substantial when compared to the average U.S. per capita health expenditure in 2000 of $4,636. In the CPC study, 26 percent of patients reported that their symptoms resulted in absenteeism from work, at an average cost of $551 over the 3 months prior to entry into the study. This equates to a mean yearly indirect cost of $2,204 per patient. Additionally, 79 percent of the CPC study participants reported being at least a little less productive while at work and attributed 50 percent of this productivity loss to their prostatitis symptoms. Twenty-two percent of the men reported having a friend or spouse help them with personal care, medical care, or activities around the house because of their prostatitis. Overall, 49 percent of the men in the CPC study reported that prostatitis disrupted their leisure time, with a 20 percent average reduction in the amount of time spent on leisure activities.

Research Priorities and Recommendations

* Create new studies or expand existing studies, such as the NAMCS or the National Health and Nutrition Examination Survey, to incorporate resource use and cost data. These studies should be longitudinal to capture long-term consequences of therapies. Data should not be limited to Medicare aged patients. This is important as research to date is largely limited by the quality of available data. In addition, current administrative datasets (e.g., Medicare) are often limited by a lack of clinical detail (e.g., symptoms severity and complications data).

* Promote the involvement of health economists, decision analysts, and health services researchers who are also urologists interested in examining decision making and health care economics. Support of T32 and other training/career development programs that promote this among graduating urology residents should be fostered. Centers of excellence for training urologic health services researchers should be established for long-term viability.

* Develop a prospective means to examine the direct and indirect costs and cost-effectiveness of contemporary treatment modalities for benign prostate disease over the long term. This can be done using administrative datasets or larger population-based cohort studies.

* Develop strategies to disseminate cost effectiveness data and teach clinicians to use therapies in a more cost-efficient manner. Physicians are generally resistant to incorporating costs in the decision-making process with their patients.

References:

1. McConnell JD, Barry MJ, Bruskewitz, R.C. et al. *Benign Prostatic Hyperplasia: Diagnosis and Treatment. Clinical Practice Guideline No. 8.* AHCPR Pub. No. 94-0582. Rockville, MD: Agency for Health Care Policy and Research, Public Health Service, U.S. Department of Health and Human Services; 1994.

2. Weis KA, Epstein RS, Huse DM, Deverka PA, Oster G. The costs of prostatectomy for benign prostatic hyperplasia. *Prostate* 1993;22(4):325-334.

3. Goluboff ET, Olsson CA. Urologists on a tightrope: coping with a changing economy. *Journal of Urology* 1994;151(1):1-4.

4. Saigal CS, Joyce G. Economic costs of benign prostatic hyperplasia in the private sector. *Journal of Urology* 2005;173(4):1309-1313.

5. Wei JT, Calhoun E, Jacobsen SJ. Urologic diseases in America project: benign prostatic hyperplasia. *Journal of Urology* 2005;173(4):1256-1261.

6. Top 200 Brand-Name Drugs By Retail Sales In 2002. *Verispan Scott-Levin.* SPA 2008. Available at: URL: http://drugtopics. modernmedicine.com/drugtopics/article/articleDetail.jsp?id=104562. Accessed March 5, 2008.

7. Wei JT, Calhoun EA, Jacobsen SJ. Benign prostatic hyperplasia. In: Litwin MS, Saigal CS, eds. *Urologic Diseases in America.* U.S. Department of Health and Human Services, National Institutes of Health, National Institute of Diabetes and Digestive and Kidney Diseases. Washington, DC: U.S. Government Printing Office, NIH Publication No. 07-5512; 2007. pp. 43-70.

8. Black L, Naslund MJ, Gilbert TD, Jr., Davis EA, Ollendorf DA. An examination of treatment patterns and costs of care among patients with benign prostatic hyperplasia. *The American Journal of Managed Care* 2006;12(4 Suppl):S99-S110.

9. McDonald H, Hux M, Brisson M, Bernard L, Nickel JC. An economic evaluation of doxazosin, finasteride and combination therapy in the treatment of benign prostatic hyperplasia. *Canadian Journal of Urology* 2004;11(4):2327-2340.

10. DiSantostefano RL, Biddle AK, Lavelle JP. The long-term cost effectiveness of treatments for benign prostatic hyperplasia. *Pharmacoeconomics* 2006;24(2):171-191.

11. McNaughton-Collins M, Joyce GF, Wise M, Pontari MA. Prostatitis. In: Litwin MS, Saigal CS, eds. *Urologic Diseases in America.* U.S. Department of Health and Human Services, National Institutes of Health, National Institute of Diabetes and Digestive and Kidney Diseases. Washington, DC: U.S. Government Printing Office, NIH Publication No. 07-5512; 2007, pp. 9-42.

12. Clemens JQ, Meenan RT, O'Keeffe Rosetti MC, Gao SY, Calhoun EA. Analysis of medical costs in men associated with prostatitis. Presented at the American Urological Association Meeting May 20-25, 2006, Atlanta, GA.

13. Turner JA, Ciol MA, Von Korff M, Rothman I, Berger RE. Healthcare use and costs of primary and secondary care patients with prostatitis. *Urology* 2004;63(6):1031-1035.

14. Calhoun EA, McNaughton CM, Pontari MA, et al. The economic impact of chronic prostatitis. *Archives of Internal Medicine* 2004;164(11):1231-1236.

The goals of therapeutic management of benign prostate disease, such as BPH and prostatitis, for the physician should be to provide long-term relief of symptoms in an objective, economical, and efficient manner without the need for recurrent procedures. How patients actually make a decision about therapy is largely unknown. BPH patients often present with LUTS then proceed in their care through watchful waiting, medical therapy, to some form of surgical therapy, usually on the basis of LUTS assessments through AUA symptom scores or IPSS. The forms of surgical therapy start with "minimally invasive" treatments, such as TUNA and TUMT, and then may advance to more formal surgical procedures, such as laser prostatectomy, TURP, or open simple prostatectomy. This amounts to a cascade of failing treatments until a prostatectomy is performed. The major therapeutic decision points are starting medication and deciding on surgical intervention. The surgical decision is usually based on "failure of medical management" (which seems to be difficult to define) or evidence of non-resolving acute urinary retention, renal insufficiency due to outlet obstruction, development of urinary tract infection, or bladder calculi.

Decision Making for BPH

The correlation of LUTS with bladder outlet obstruction (BOO) is obvious when the patient goes into urinary retention. However, what is not correlated are symptoms and degree of obstruction prior to urinary retention. Physicians may use decreasing flow rates or increasing post-void residuals as evidence of BOO; however, these tests are unreliable due to considerable variance in their results. Urodynamic testing with outcome prediction also have been shown not to correlate well. The other problem is that a number of men present with urinary retention and it is discovered that their bladder cannot generate pressure to provide micturition (i.e., voiding). This may be idiopathic or due to neurological disorders or diabetes. Identification of this problem is generally not made until after the bladder can no longer generate pressure. The failure of bladder function may be permanent and depending on the patients circumstances, leads to some permanent form of catheter dependent drainage.

Currently, it appears that most therapeutic decisions are driven by worsening symptoms affecting QOL.

Unfortunately, there are no reliable objective measures of BOO except the obvious end-points described earlier to determine the degree of BOO necessitating a change from medical therapy to surgery. Most BPH management now occurs in the family practitioners office with little or no testing while the patients are taking medication. Therefore, the decision of "failure of medical management" may be delayed or not made by a urologist.

Confounding current BPH management is developing evidence that irritative symptoms may be related to bladder overactivity and the combined use of antimuscarinic therapies with alpha-blocker or 5-alpha-reductase therapies to relieve symptoms. Symptoms of overactive bladder (OAB) also seem to have an impact on QOL and at the present time, it is difficult to objectively separate OAB and BOO symptoms.

Ultimately, therapeutic decisions are made between the patient and physician mostly based on symptoms and QOL, which may not relate to the degree of bladder outlet obstruction or loss of urologic function. Treatment modalities progress through medical therapy with increasing medication until the patient decides that surgery is required or the patient has objective surgical indications. At this point, surgical interventions increase in invasiveness until a prostatectomy is performed, which will generally give long-term relief of obstructive symptoms, but not necessarily irritative symptoms like frequency.

Decision Making for Prostatitis

One of the first challenges in clinical care is to distinguish CP/CPPS from BPH. This is made by recognizing the presence of pain. A major decision here is whether the pain is from causes different than those that result solely in LUTS, thus suggesting the possibility of CP/CPPS, or if the pain represents a more severe manifestation of the same pathophysiology underlying LUTS.

Once CP/CPPS is diagnosed, the first line of treatment is usually a course of antibiotics. There are data that support an empiric course of antibiotics for men with CP/CPPS even without a documented infection (though overuse of antibiotics remains a quality of care issue in need of attention). However, the optimal duration of antibiotic treatment leading to benefits that outweigh risks is unknown. Alpha-blockers are commonly used following antibiotics, though the optimal length of treatment for CP/CPPS is also unclear. Also, unknown is the optimal order of front line medical treatments. Correlation of treatment response to known past medical risk factors needs to be studied. The role of neuroimaging appears to be a pressing issue, given the current thinking that CP/CPPS may involve alterations in the central nervous system in some men.

Research Priorities and Recommendations

- Correlate treatment response to known past medical risk factors in men with CP/CPPS.
- Assess the utility of neuroimaging in evaluating CP/CPPS.
- Examine contemporary practice patterns for new therapies and develop clinical educational aids for decision making for patients and clinicians. Little is known about decision making for proceeding to

surgical and minimally invasive therapies. Given the wealth of options, it is not uncommon to have patients "run the gamut" of treatments ranging from medical management to MIST to surgery.
- Engage medical students to study BPH and prostatitis through formal urology curricula.
- Use public health relationships to establish and develop educational tools to assess which men understand benign prostate diseases and to educate men on the differences between benign prostate disease and prostate cancer.
- Determine the current knowledge level of men about BPH, prostatitis, and their therapies.
- Implement high-level evidence into decision making. There is a need to develop and disseminate physician- and patient-centric decision aids that address therapy options and outcomes, including side effects and costs.
- Determine the influence of costs/reimbursements on management decisions related to benign prostate disease.

High-Priority Recommendations

- Develop classification schemes for benign prostate disease based on new insights into underlying etiology.
- Develop data and tissue resources that contain well-characterized population-based information necessary for investigation of risk factors, natural history, etiologic mechanisms, QOL, quality of care, and decision making for benign prostate disease.
- Communicate the importance of rigorous clinical research methodologies when applied in the basic, clinical, and population-based settings.

- Ensure that high-quality study designs are used to generate and test hypotheses of key significance to benign prostatic disease.
- Disseminate clinical trial findings, medical and surgical therapies, evidence-based medicine, and health-related QOL measures into clinical practice.
- Train and mentor epidemiologists, health services researchers, clinical investigators, and students interested in study of benign prostate disease.

III. Translational Opportunities

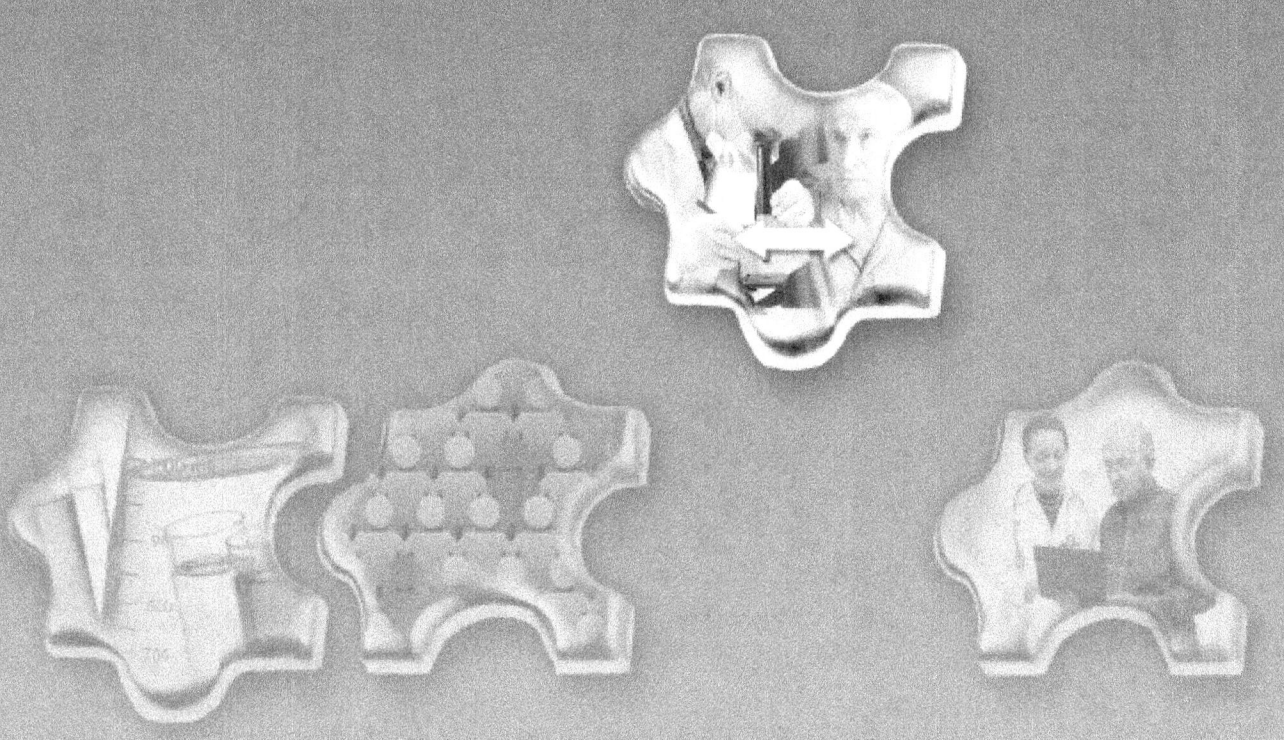

Mission Statement

The primary goal of translational research focused on benign prostatic diseases is to advance the clinical care of patients suffering from these disorders. Translation research involves the bidirectional movement of concepts between the basic research laboratory and the clinical setting, using technologies to better define and stratify clinical populations, examining observations from the clinic in the laboratory, and developing resources that facilitate the flow of findings between the laboratory and the clinical setting (Figure 1). This Translational Opportunities section integrates basic science, epidemiological/ population-based studies, and clinical science studies to promote important directions and common resources for translational research. Specific areas of interest involve the identification and interface of novel disease markers and therapeutic approaches.

*T*ranslational research involves the bidirectional movement of key scientific concepts and findings between the laboratory and the clinical setting with the ultimate goal of facilitating the understanding of and prevention and treatment of disease.

Scientific inquiry into benign diseases of the prostate and related syndromes has evolved into two distinct areas, that of basic science and clinical science. Unfortunately, there are too few efforts that bridge the gap between those studying basic disease mechanisms and those who are actively involved in patient-oriented investigations and treatment. In many cases, basic scientists may be evaluating mechanisms that, while important to science, have little or no clinical relevance and clinical scientists may make observations that are never examined in the laboratory.

Too few findings related to benign prostate diseases and related syndromes have been translated either from the laboratory to the clinic or from the clinic back to the laboratory. This may be attributed to a number of issues, including the fact that few new ideas relating to the basic mechanisms of disease pathology have been put forth. In addition, the patient populations are, in general, poorly defined. This makes studies of benign prostate disease difficult. Furthermore, there is insufficient application of new and novel technologies to the study and treatment of these diseases and few well-characterized resources or specimen banks are available with which to move studies from the bench to the bedside. Finally, there are too few established investigators and multidisciplinary teams addressing these concepts. Clearly, there is a need for improved translational research in the area of benign prostate disease.

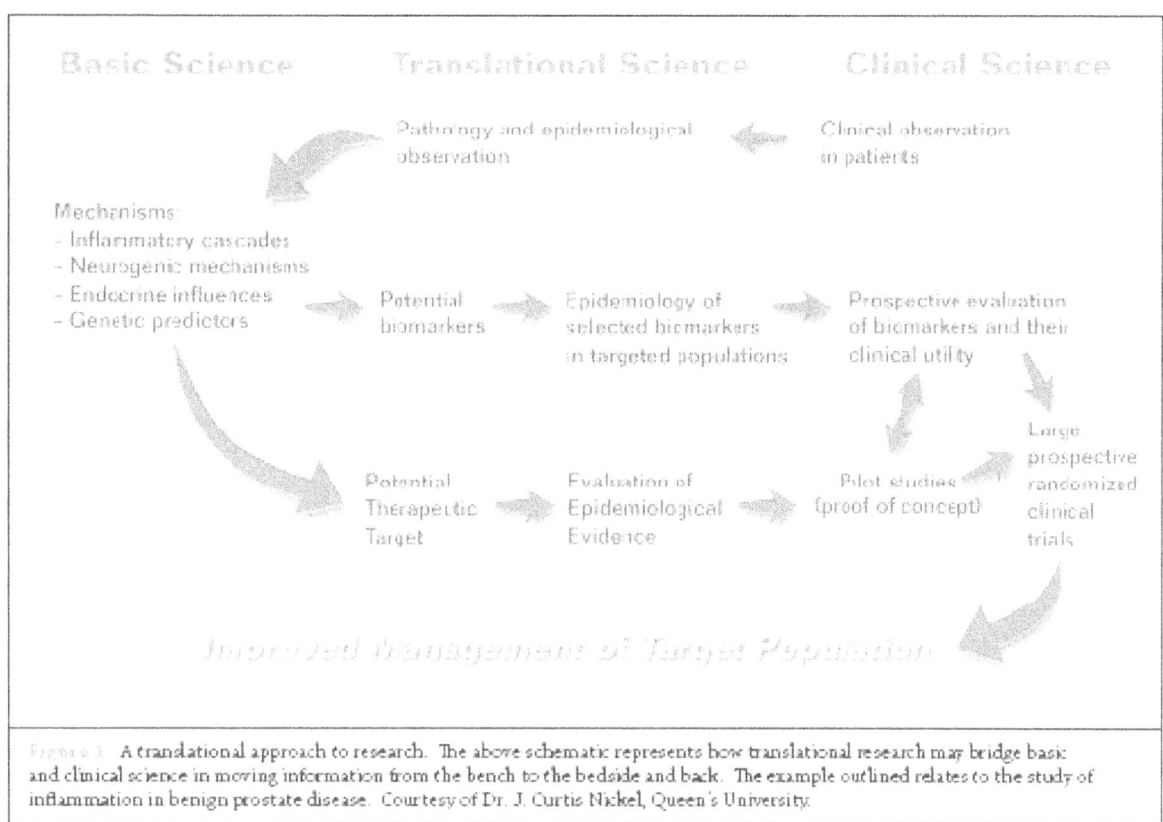

Figure 1. A translational approach to research. The above schematic represents how translational research may bridge basic and clinical science in moving information from the bench to the bedside and back. The example outlined relates to the study of inflammation in benign prostate disease. Courtesy of Dr. J. Curtis Nickel, Queen's University.

22. Overall Infrastructure Needs

The translation of new ideas between the laboratory and the clinical setting is perhaps the biggest need facing the field of benign prostate disease. Specific priorities for emphasized research areas are detailed in the following chapters. Several general recommendations for fostering translational research are as follows:

- Identify and encourage new investigators and the establishment of working basic scientist-clinician research relationships. Specific infrastructure needs include:
  - Providing incentives to promote and encourage the clinical and/or basic scientist who is interested in a translational approach to studying benign prostate disease.

  - Providing events/methods to educate and encourage basic scientist-clinician research collaborations (e.g., workshops, novel funding mechanisms, and newer "center of excellence" based approaches).

- Develop standardized, clinically significant prostate disease/syndrome definitions that can be characterized by measurable phenotypic features. Addressing this need also may help to address the above need.

- Define commonalities (e.g., pathological, clinical, and molecular) that are shared between clinical syndromes (e.g., benign prostatic hyperplasia [BPH], chronic pelvic pain, prostatitis, etc.). A specific infrastructure need is to organize a consensus conference on standardization of classification for benign prostate disease and related syndromes.

23. Serum and Tissue Biorepositories for Prostatic Disease

One of the biggest obstacles to translational research in benign prostatic disease and related syndromes has been the lack of suitable biopsy tissue, urine, and sera in sufficient quantities to objectively monitor histologic and/or molecular changes associated with disease progression or therapeutic intervention. Most biomarker and histologic research today is performed on human tissues and sera obtained at surgery or biopsy at individual institutions using protocols and methods that are standard for that institution. These protocols and methods often differ from institution to institution, as do the characteristics of the patients and disease in question. Therefore, a marker that is found to have clinical utility in one institutional study may not be validated when applied to another institution's samples. Differences in how tissues and/or sera are handled from the moment they are removed from the body to testing may account for a large part of these discrepancies. Recent network initiatives to form multi-institutional specimen banks using standardized protocols across the individual centers have attempted to address some of these problems.[1,2]

Differences in the scope of disease and definitions of advanced or progressive disease between different

institutions also pose a problem for translational studies. For instance, BPH investigators at different institutions may define advanced BPH in different ways, such as American Urological Association symptom score versus the need for surgery. Because tissue is usually obtained only at surgery, finding suitable controls for comparative studies is very problematic. Furthermore, differences in which pathological changes are recorded for benign tissues collected ultimately affect the utility of the banked tissue for research. Finally, there needs to be a means of identifying and distributing proper tissue and other biological samples to research investigators for research use, particularly in times of increasing institutional review board and Health Insurance Portability and Accountability Act constraints.

Recent efforts to establish tissue, serum, and urine biorepositories from large multi-center clinical trials have created unique and opportune resources for translational research. An important byproduct of the Medical Therapy of Prostate Symptoms (MTOPS) trial was the establishment of large specimen banks of both biopsy tissue and serum obtained from patients at various time points during the course of the trial. Specimen banks have been most commonly created for malignancies whose initial therapy is surgical resection of the tumor. The creation of a specimen bank for primarily benign prostate tissue (with concomitant serum specimens) offers a unique opportunity to study the pathways of benign prostate disease, the inter-relationships of benign and malignant diseases, as well as common and unique biomarkers for disease detection and progression. The serial collections of tissue and serum also allow a more precise study of the impact of study drugs on benign prostate disease.

The MTOPS specimen archive has several key advantages over single institution biorepositories that are characteristic of a well-conceived archive with great utility. First, the tissue was harvested from patients throughout the United States and processed centrally using a uniform protocol. This ensures that information obtained from subsequent biomarker studies is comparable across the entire specimen cohort and not adversely effected by time of fixation, type of fixative, method of staining, etc. This also assured that no tissue was wasted during processing, thereby allowing for ample material for follow-up studies. Second, the biopsies were read by a central pathologist for more uniformity of diagnoses and meticulously recorded as to the histopathologic features on each biopsy. Serum samples from every patient blood draw also were frozen in 0.5 mL aliquots and can be paired with biopsy findings. Again, a central laboratory performed all serum tests for Prostate Specific Antigen (PSA), hormone levels, etc. Moreover, the tissue and serum was archived in an appropriate central facility (Figure 2) with great care taken to preserve and conserve specimens for the purposes of future research. Finally, detailed clinical followup is available on all MTOPS patients allowing for the correlation of observed cellular characteristics (e.g., biomarker expression, morphology, etc.) with clinical outcomes.

In the case of the MTOPS tissue samples, biopsies of prostate transition zone and peripheral zone tissue were obtained on 1,081 randomized patients, and baseline histology and morphometric values were established. Biopsies were repeated on the same randomized patients at 1-year and end-of-study (5 years) to assess changes in histology and morphometric values. The MTOPS repository contains more than 3,000 formalin-fixed, paraffin-embedded multicore biopsies, and approximately 6,000 unfixed frozen biopsy cores. All MTOPS specimens were integrated into a Microsoft SQL server database

that contains relevant information on collection and characteristics of specimens. The biorepository has served as an integral component of the NIDDK's MTOPS Prostate Samples Analysis (MPSA) Consortium.[3] To our knowledge, this is the only repository that exists for benign prostatic disease in which serial serum and tissue samples were collected from a multi-institutional trial in a uniform manner and linked with clinical data.

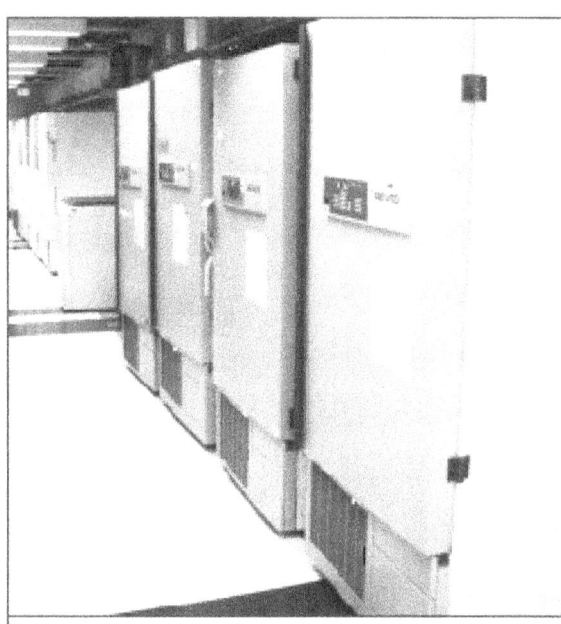

Figure 2. Standard biosample storage facility for the long-term archiving of samples (e.g., biopsy, serum, and urine) at low temperature. Courtesy of Dr. M. Scott Lucia, University of Colorado.

Research Priorities and Recommendations

- Capitalize on opportunities to collect, characterize, and archive sera, urine, and/or tissue during patient management and clinical trials using standardized protocols and definitions.
- Encourage standardized institutional archiving using:
    - Uniform protocols and database fields (as an example, see http://biospecimens.cancer.gov/global/pdfs/NCI_Best_Practices_060507.pdf).
    - Network and/or pool archived samples between institutions.
    - Create common platform pools (e.g., pools of samples of specific utility for serum/tissue array methodologies).
- Establish funding mechanisms for biorepository efforts.

References:

1. Gohagan JK, Prorok PC, Hayes RB, Kramer BS. The Prostate, Lung, Colorectal and Ovarian (PLCO) Cancer Screening Trial of the National Cancer Institute: history, organization, and status. *Controlled Clinical Trials* 2000;21(6 Suppl):251S–272S.

2. Melamed J, Datta MW, Becich MJ, et al. The cooperative prostate cancer tissue resource: a specimen and data resource for cancer researchers. *Clinical Cancer Research* 2004;10(14):4614–4621.

3. Mullins C, Lucia MS, Hayward SW, et al. A comprehensive approach toward novel serum biomarkers for benign prostatic hyperplasia: the MPSA Consortium. *Journal of Urology* 2008;179(4):1243–1256.

24. Database Studies and Informatics

Our understanding of benign prostatic diseases has been hampered by a lack of extensive epidemiology and population-based studies. In fact, there are very few publications in this area that relate to the complex problems associated with these benign diseases. However, some valuable resources do exist that can be used to mine existing epidemiological data and, thus provide insights into the etiology of these diseases and for the development of prevention and therapeutic strategies. For example, there are a number of databases that may be used to evaluate factors related to the development of benign prostate disease and related treatment outcomes. Sources of data include clinical trials, observational studies, and surveys, including MTOPS, the Chronic Prostatitis Collaborative Research Network, *Urologic Diseases in America*, and the National Health and Nutrition and Examination Survey. The effort of individuals equipped with the appropriate scientific tools is required to fully decipher these disease sets to determine potentially valuable information that can be translated into novel therapeutic approaches, prevention strategies, and markers for disease.

In addition to the existing data resources, there is a need to develop new database resources and enhance ongoing resources. These data sets should be built from ongoing and planned clinical trials for new treatment strategies for relevant diseases. In addition, both the placebo groups, as well as the treatment populations, from clinical trials focused on prostate cancer should be studied. For example, the Prostate Cancer Prevention Trial and current dutasteride prostate cancer prevention trials involved the use of 5-alpha-reductase inhibitors to inhibit the development of prostate cancer. Regardless of the results of these trials in influencing the development and/or progression of prostate cancer, these studies represent unique opportunities to examine the natural history of benign prostatic diseases.

Research Priorities and Recommendations

- Describe, characterize, and advertise the databases for prostatic disease that currently exist (e.g., bioinformatics networks).
- Search current databases for:
  - Identification of risk factors for benign prostate disease for the purpose of developing screening and preventive measures.
  - Assessment of prognostic factors for clinical outcome.
  - Evaluation of longitudinal changes in function and quality of life for treatments and natural history patients.
  - Evaluation of the potential correlations between markers of inflammation and clinical outcomes.
- Develop a systematic approach to prospective collection of data on benign prostate disease.
- Improve public awareness of prostate disease symptoms and potential interventions to alleviate symptoms and treat benign prostate disease.

Infrastructure Needs

- Promote opportunities for secondary analyses of existing databases.
- Promote common data elements and mechanisms for data collection for future databases (e.g., web-based).

BPH is characterized by prostatic enlargement due to nodular expansion of the prostate periurethral or transition zones. The first researcher to systematically describe BPH subdivided its lesions into fibrous, leiomyomatous (predominantly composed of smooth muscle), fibroadenamatous (fibrous and glandular components), and fibromyoadenomatous (fibrous, smooth muscular, and glandular components) types.[1] This categorical description has not changed substantially over the last 50 years, but from a clinical standpoint it is of limited utility. Conceptually, the nodules of BPH are composed of glandular, smooth muscle, and fibrous elements in variable proportions. As these nodules grow in size, they display complex changes in their cellular components (Figure 3). The glands in BPH nodules often contain intraglandular papillae or complex cribriform arrangements indicating some degree of epithelial hyperplasia. In mixed glandular-stromal nodules, there is concomitant surrounding stromal hyperplasia composed of fibroblastic and smooth muscular cell types. Nodules may even be exclusively stromal in nature with variable composition of fibroblastic and smooth muscular cell types. In small stromal nodules that develop in the periurethral region, the mesenchyme often appears similar to embryonal mesenchyme with high concentrations of acid mucopolysaccharide in the matrix.[2] As nodules become larger, vessel density increases and glandular elements become more prominent.

The importance of relative nodule composition with respect to clinical presentation and progression is unclear. Studies using computer-assisted image analysis on the relative tissue composition of baseline biopsies from men with symptomatic BPH recruited for the MTOPS trial indicate that prostate volume and symptom progression in BPH correlate with a relative percent volume increase in the stromal (i.e., smooth muscle and fibrous tissue) compartment of the transition zone.[3] Although local growth factors are certainly implicated, the precise nature of the apparent epithelial-stromal interactions is still largely unknown. Furthermore, the nature of the stimulus for cellular growth is unknown. For example, are the epithelial and/or stromal cells responding to a pathologic environmental stimulus or are they responding inappropriately to a physiologic stimulus? The potential for translating these findings into better clinical diagnosis or prediction of clinical outcomes is an area of important future study.

In addition to changes in stromal/epithelial composition, inflammation is a very common histological finding in patients with symptomatic BPH. Although it is generally recognized that acute and chronic inflammation frequently occur in association with BPH nodules, the inter-relationships of these disease processes are poorly defined. The question remains as to whether inflammation plays a causal role in BPH or is a result of BPH. The prostate in general is susceptible to infiltration by lymphocytes and macrophages, with prevalence seeming to increase with age.[4] Compared to normal tissue, BPH specimens have increased infiltration of inflammatory cells, including CD3+ T-lymphocytes, CD11c+ macrophages, and CD20+ B-lymphocytes.[5] In the MTOPS trial, the risk of acute urinary retention (AUR) due to BPH was greater in men with inflammation on baseline biopsies compared to those without inflammation on their biopsies (2.4 versus 0.6 percent, p = 0.003).[6] There also was a trend towards increased overall clinical (largely symptomatic) progression in men with inflammation on biopsy compared to those without inflammation (21.0 versus 13.2 percent, p = 0.08). Although suggestive that chronic inflammation may play a role in symptom progression in BPH, the mechanistic role of inflammation in prostatic disease development and progression still remains to be elucidated. This represents another area of study with great translational potential.

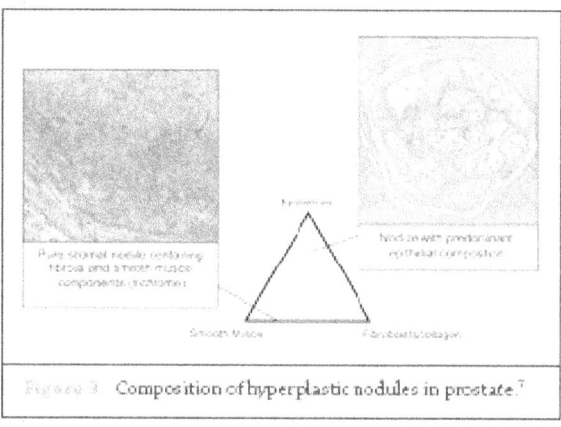

Figure 3. Composition of hyperplastic nodules in prostate.[7]

- Determine if histologic changes (e.g., inflammatory, composition, angiogenesis) correlate with disease severity and risk of progression in BPH/lower urinary tract symptoms (LUTS).
- Determine the utility of prostate biopsy and immunohistochemistry studies/findings in the evaluation of progression, risk, and treatment response for BPH/LUTS.
- Determine whether treatments that target inflammation, angiogenesis, or both inhibit the development of BPH nodules and alter the

pathology on biopsy (e.g., histopathology or immunohistochemistry changes).

Infrastructure Needs

- Capture biorepository materials from men with BPH that are linked with databases with complete clinical data are mandatory for the success of the above-described translational research. Biopsy tissues from men in BPH clinical trials for whom detailed recording of progression events is performed are ideal (such as was collected for the MTOPS trial).

References:

1. Franks LM. Benign nodular hyperplasia of the prostate; a review. *Annals of the Royal College of Surgeons of England* 1953;14(2):92–106.

2. Bierhoff E, Walljasper U, Hofmann D, Vogel J, Wernert N, Pfeifer U. Morphological analogies of fetal prostate stroma and stromal nodules in BPH. *Prostate* 1997;31(4):234–240.

3. Lucia MS, Noble WD, McConnell JD, Roehrborn CG, Kusek JW, Nyberg LM. Tissue composition analysis in baseline transition zone biopsies in the MTOPS trial. *Journal of Urology* 2005;173(4):388 Abstr. no. 1432.

4. Kohnen PW, Drach GW. Patterns of inflammation in prostatic hyperplasia: a histologic and bacteriologic study. *Journal of Urology* 1979;121(6):755–760.

5. Steiner G, Gessl A, Kramer G, Schollhammer A, Forster O, Marberger M. Phenotype and function of peripheral and prostatic lymphocytes in patients with benign prostatic hyperplasia. *Journal of Urology* 1994;151(2):480–484.

6. Roehrborn CG, Kaplan SA, Noble WD, et al. The impact of acute or chronic inflammation in baseline biopsy on the risk of clinical progression of BPH: Results from the MTOPS study. *Journal of Urology* 2005;173(4):346 Abstr. no. 1277.

7. Lucia MS and Lambert JR. Growth factors in benign prostatic hyperplasia: basic science implications. *Current Prostate Reports* 2007;5:78–84.

26. Biomarkers

Unfortunately, there are very few molecular or cellular markers (i.e., biomarkers) available for detailed studies of prostate biology and associated benign prostatic diseases. Historically, the major biomarkers studied in prostate biology are PSA and its isoforms, prostate specific membrane antigen, and the androgen receptor. Recent studies using both proteomic and genomic technologies have revealed particular biomarkers associated with disease processes (some of these are described below). However, one traditional limitation in the development of biomarkers for benign prostate disease has been the lack of a good classification system for prostate disease types.

Recently, potential serum markers for BPH have been identified and tested through a number of strategies. Biomarkers like BPSA (i.e., the BPH isoform of PSA) have resulted from efforts taking advantage of the properties of PSA to define an isoform that may be associated with BPH/LUTS.[1] BPSA is being studied as a biomarker with potential to provide clinical discrimination between BPH/LUTS and other prostate

diseases, including prostate cancer. By using genomic profiling to identify potential biomarkers, it has become apparent that not all BPH/LUTS is created the same. The biological discrimination between histologic and highly symptomatic BPH has been dramatic.[2] Such studies have led to the identification of biomarkers such as JM-27 (Figure 4). The transcript for JM-27 was initially identified as highly specific for symptomatic BPH (i.e., clinical BPH or LUTS). The JM-27 protein is a member of the cancer-testis antigen family. Recent reports have demonstrated that antibodies raised against this protein can detect symptomatic BPH in both tissue and serum samples.[3,4] Further JM-27 validation studies are ongoing.

The MPSA Program established by the NIDDK has provided the opportunity to identify a number of potential markers associated with BPH and specifically with symptomatic disease.[5] This program developed a logical progression pathway through which biomarkers of benign prostatic diseases may be developed and validated. Using diverse expertise and methodological approaches, this effort has identified a number of novel candidate biomarkers, some of which are now being validated using the MTOPS biosample archive. The sample sets collected as part of the MTOPS trial provide a rich resource validating biomarkers relative to clinical utility in assessing the disease course of BPH/LUTS. One of the limits of this sample set is that it consists of only serum (and biopsy) samples. Urine, semen, and/or prostatic secretion samples are not available. Although considerable interest in serum exists, additional sample sets consisting of a wider range of biosamples (e.g., urine, semen, prostatic secretions, etc.) also linked to clinical data need to be established and validated to facilitate the identification of biomarkers and to translate these findings into clinically relevant prevention or treatment tools.

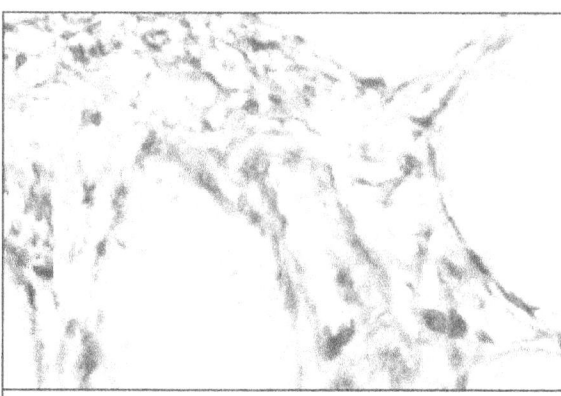
Figure 3. Immunohistochemical staining of JM-27 in the prostate.

In addition to fluid-based markers that most often are considered, additional markers include tissue-based biomarkers, as well as anatomical markers derived from imaging modalities. In the area of tissue-based markers, little has been done to characterize markers of clinical utility. Similarly, the area of imaging of the prostate and/or bladder to study prostatitis or BPH/LUTS has been largely ignored.

Research Priorities and Recommendations

- Serum and/or Urine-Based Biomarkers:
  - Develop serum, semen, and/or urine-based biomarkers that have utility for identifying progressive benign prostate disease.
  - Identify serum, semen, and/or urine-based biomarkers that can identify men at risk of developing symptomatic BPH/LUTS.
  - Identify biomarkers for distinguishing various etiologic mechanisms of benign prostate disease, such as for category III prostatitis (i.e., chronic prostatitis and chronic pelvic pain syndrome [CP/CPPS]).
  - Translate findings from biomarker studies to identify novel therapeutic targets for development of clinical treatments.
- Genomic and/or Proteomic Signatures:
  - Develop specific genomic and/or proteomic signature profiles for: (a) various forms of prostatitis, (b) progressive BPH, and (c) benign versus cancerous disease.
  - Translate findings from molecular/genomic profiles to identification of novel therapeutic targets.
- Tissue-Based Biomarkers:
  - Develop tissue-based biomarkers that can predict risk of progressive/severe BPH based on biopsy.
  - Define the potential role of tissue biomarkers for defining prostatitis (e.g., CP/CPPS) syndromes.
  - Develop tissue microarrays that can easily be applied to new biomarkers as they are developed.
- Imaging Modalities:
  - Develop imaging approaches to assess disease severity/risk of progression based on biomarker studies (e.g., metabolomics).

Infrastructure Needs

- Develop a standard set of samples (e.g., serum, urine, semen, and/or prostatic secretions and tissue) that can be evaluated at different stages of biomarker development to allow investigators to determine the potential utility of their biomarkers.
- Provide incentives to promote leading investigators in biomarker development to ask questions related to benign prostate disease.
- Take advantage of the extensive work conducted on prostate cancer biomarkers, some of which may be applied in studies of benign prostate disease.

References

1. Linton HJ, Marks LS, Millar LS, Knott CL, Rittenhouse HG, Mikolajczyk SD. Benign prostate-specific antigen (BPSA) in serum is increased in benign prostate disease. *Clinical Chemistry* 2003;49(2):253–259.

2. Prakash K, Pirozzi G, Elashoff M, et al. Symptomatic and asymptomatic benign prostatic hyperplasia: molecular differentiation by using microarrays. *Proceedings of the National Academy of Sciences of the United States of America* 2002;99(11):7598–7603.

3. Cannon GW, Mullins C, Lucia MS, et al. A preliminary study of JM-27: a serum marker that can specifically identify men with symptomatic benign prostatic hyperplasia. *Journal of Urology* 2007;177(2):610–614.

4. Shah US, Arlotti J, Dhir R, et al. Androgen regulation of JM-27 is associated with the diseased prostate. *Journal of Andrology* 2004;25(4):618–624.

5. Mullins C, Lucia MS, Hayward SW, et al. A comprehensive approach toward novel serum biomarkers for benign prostatic hyperplasia: the MPSA Consortium. *Journal of Urology* 2008;Epub ahead of print.

27. Genetics and Epigenetics

Genetics

There appears to be a genetic component to BPH. This is supported by studies showing an increased risk for BPH in men with a family history of the disease and higher concordance rates in monozygotic twins. However, the genetic basis is likely to be polygenic, similar to prostate cancer, and thus involving many different genes with small individual contributions. There are a handful of studies that have examined specific gene variants in relation to BPH, most with inconclusive or negative findings. The majority of genetic studies involving BPH are done in studies using BPH as the benign comparator to prostate cancer. There is a need for gene-identification studies that compare BPH with normal tissue.

Familial genetic studies have long been the standard for identifying genetic causes of many diseases. However, these studies have some serious limitations, including limited availability of eligible participants due to small family sizes, a problem that is exacerbated when studying prostatic diseases that have late onset and are gender specific.

Genetic association studies that look for associations between genetic polymorphisms (e.g., individual single nucleotide polymorphisms and/or gene haplotypes) and disease in unrelated groups may be a better methodological fit for studying benign prostatic diseases. These studies have more power than family studies for the identification of small effects. However, it is often difficult to repeat findings in subsequent studies. This may be due to differing case-control definitions and selection criteria, small sample sizes, and different ethnic composition (i.e., population stratification) of the samples. Population stratification may confound the results of some prostatic disease association studies because the incidence of these diseases may vary by ethnicity. If a polymorphism also has different frequencies by race, it may appear to be associated with the disease when there is really no true causal relationship. It is important for genetic association studies that examine different ethnicities to control for potential confounding by matching cases and controls on race/ethnicity or by measuring racial admixture using genetic markers.

Looking for small genetic effects is more difficult in the face of the differing definitions for benign prostatic diseases. Genetic studies may not be productive until standardized, non-subjective disease definitions are developed. Properly executed, such studies have great potential for identification of genetic markers for diseases that may translate into improved clinical diagnosis or practice.

Epigenetics

Epigenetics refers to features of chromatin and DNA modifications that are stable during growth and through multiple rounds of cell division but that do not involve changes in the underlying primary sequence of the DNA.[1] Aberrant modifications to the DNA or histone core of chromatin play crucial roles in normal processes and disease development (despite identical genomic composition) and are ultimately reversible. Thus, these are potentially ideal targets for therapeutic intervention.

Mechanisms of epigenetic modification in human disease have been extensively studied, yet therapeutic strategies targeting these mechanisms have lagged far behind. The demethlyating agent, 5-aza-2'-deoxycytidine (5-aza), remains the focus of clinical therapy in epigenetics in various diseases. The synergistic activities of histone deacetylase inhibitors and DNA methyltransferase inhibitors have gained recent support.[2]

The vast majority of or epigenetic research in prostate disease has been fixated on malignant processes. Much less research has been focused on benign disease and pathologies. Epigenetic modifications are likely associated with benign processes such as BPH and inflammatory disease; however, much more work needs to be done in this area.

Research Priorities and Recommendations

* Promote studies to examine epigenetic changes in men with BPH and prostatitis (e.g., CP/CPPS) for the purpose of establishing expression patterns and potential biomarkers and therapeutic targets.

References:

1. Bird A. Perceptions of epigenetics. *Nature* 2007;447(7143):396–398.

2. Zhu WG, Otterson GA. The interaction of histone deacetylase inhibitors and DNA methyltransferase inhibitors in the treatment of human cancer cells. *Current Medicinal Chemistry Anticancer Agents* 2003;3(3):187–199.

High-Priority Recommendations

* Develop standardized clinically significant benign prostate disease/syndrome definitions that may be characterized by measurable phenotypic features.
* Define commonalities (e.g., pathological, clinical, and molecular) that are shared between clinical syndromes (e.g., BPH, pelvic pain, prostatitis, etc.).
* Encourage standardized institutional archiving using:
  – Uniform protocols and database fields.
  – Networking and/or pooling with other institutions.
  – Creation of common platform pools (serum/tissue arrays).
* Determine whether treatments that target inflammation, angiogenesis, or both inhibit the development of BPH nodules and alter the pathology on biopsy (using histopathology or immunohistochemistry measurements).

* Investigate the relationship between histological changes with disease severity and risk for progression of BPH/LUTS.
* Develop and identify serum, semen and/or urine-based biomarkers, as well as genomic/proteomic signatures that can identify progressive BPH, identify men at risk of developing symptomatic BPH, distinguishing various etiologic mechanisms of prostatitis, and be used to identify novel therapeutic targets.

IV. Clinical Sciences

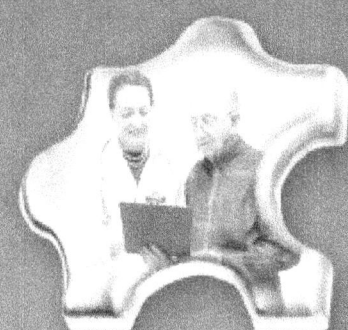

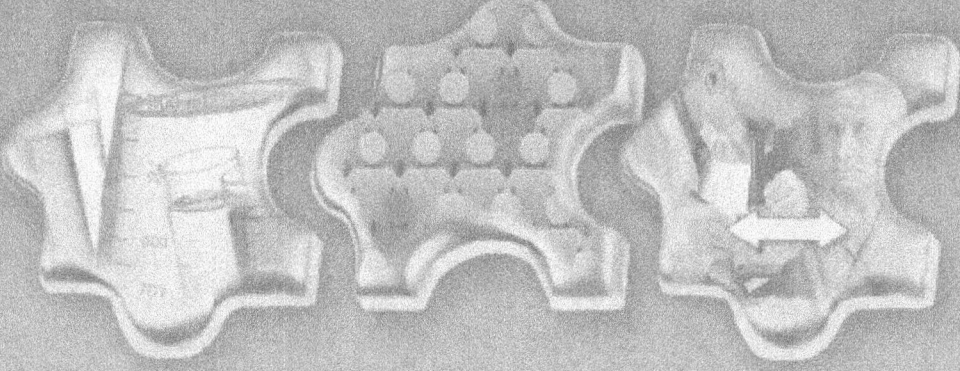

Mission Statement

This section intends to develop a prioritized list of recommendations and priorities for clinical research related to benign disorders associated with the prostate (e.g., benign prostatic hyperplasia, prostatitis, and chronic prostatitis/ chronic pelvic pain syndrome), broadly defined lower urinary tract symptoms, and general male pelvic health-related diseases. This section also makes recommendations for improving infrastructure needed to facilitate clinical research, including that needed to conduct and monitor clinical trials.

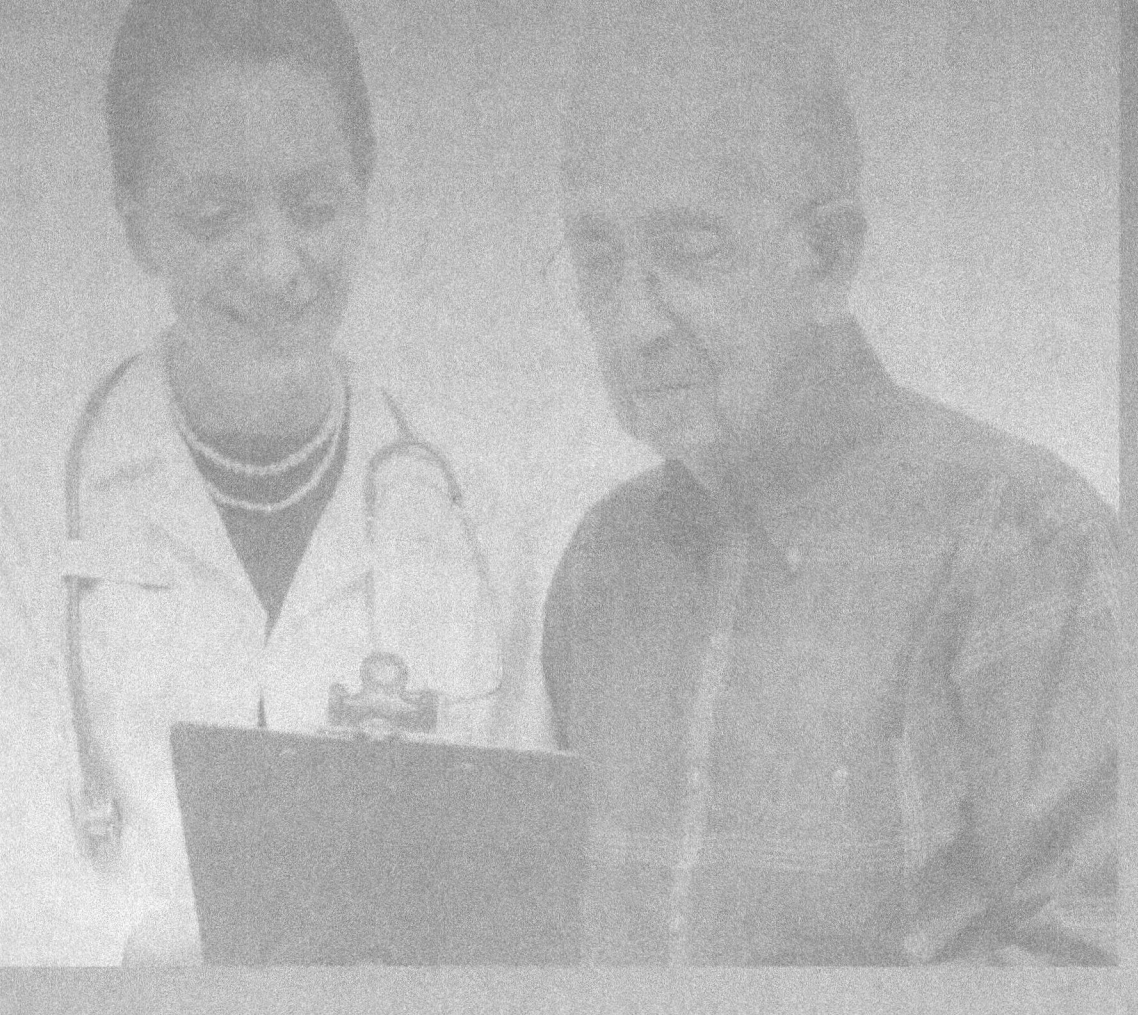

Educational/Layperson Summary

Benign prostate disease is a significant health issue for men all over the world. Two especially common benign prostate disorders are benign prostatic hyperplasia (BPH) and prostatitis. BPH, also referred to as an enlarged prostate, can be associated with diverse symptoms affecting urination and may result in significant impairment of quality of life (QOL) as men age. Another common benign prostate disorder is prostatitis. Prostatitis is characterized by pain in the pelvic area and/or infection, often in combination with problems urinating, and can severely affect men of all ages.

There are many research questions in our study of benign prostate disease that remain largely unanswered and to date, no generally useful treatments exist for these common disorders. In addition, physicians are unable to accurately diagnose and determine the severity of benign prostate disease due to the lack of reliable and consistent methods for assessing disease state and response to treatment. Addressing these deficiencies will require a cooperative effort by a diverse group of scientists. New studies must be designed to better define these diseases and identify potential treatments. This will also require more consistent and reproducible clinical trial designs to assess disease prevention, progression of disease, and responses to therapy. Clinical areas in need of increased research include development of improved methods to assess disease; testing of new drug therapies; testing of plants and other natural sources of potential drugs; assessment of behavioral and lifestyle changes, including diet and exercise; and alternative therapies to surgery, including minimally invasive therapies.

Scientific Topics/Areas of Research

28. Defining the Clinical Phenotype: Definitions and Their Importance

BPH and LUTS

Voiding symptoms in men have traditionally been thought of as secondary to an enlarged prostate, such as those symptoms associated with BPH. Men with storage and voiding symptoms were said to suffer from "prostatism." Our understanding of the etiology of voiding symptoms has, however, evolved over the past 25 years. Urodynamic studies delineated multiple etiologies for voiding symptoms, such as detrusor overactivity, impaired bladder contractility, sensory urgency, and bladder outlet obstruction. Because of a lack of consistent association between symptoms and underlying prostate pathophysiology, the term prostatism was felt to be misleading, as it wrongly focused on the prostate as the source of the symptoms. In response, the term lower urinary tract symptoms (LUTS) was proposed as an umbrella term for storage, voiding, and post-micturition (i.e., after voiding) symptoms. Indeed, LUTS is sometimes divided into three symptom subcategories: storage, voiding, and postmicturition. However, each set of symptoms is interdependent and most men with disease have a mixture of symptoms. Therefore, a strict division of LUTS into subgroups is not possible.

The subgrouping of LUTS patients is further complicated by the fact that at least four common voiding disorders increase in prevalence with age and can coexist with LUTS. Detrusor overactivity (sometimes referred to as an overactive bladder), nocturnal polyuria (i.e., excessive night-time voiding volumes), prostatic obstruction, and detrusor underactivity are all age related. The precise relationship between these conditions and whether there is a common etiology or pathophysiological factors remain key areas of current and future research. There are data to suggest that adrenergic antagonists, thought to work on the bladder outlet to reduce voiding symptoms, also may affect storage symptoms. Similarly, there is much current work investigating phosphodiesterase type 5 (PDE-5) inhibitors, usually used for erectile dysfunction (ED), for the treatment of LUTS. Furthermore, emerging data show that antimuscarinic drug therapy for men is safe, even when the man has a prostatic obstruction. These studies suggest that it is reasonable to take a longer term, holistic view of BPH/LUTS and not rush into surgical treatment for this disorder.

Chronic Prostatitis (CP)/Chronic Pelvic Pain Syndrome (CPPS)

Another major benign prostate disorder is CP/CPPS. Prostatitis may be subdivided into four different conditions, based on symptoms and presence of pathogenic infection, with CP/CPPS representing category III prostatitis. CP/CPPS is characterized by pelvic pain, variable irritative and obstructive voiding symptoms, and variable sexual dysfunction in the absence of an identified pathogen. There is considerable overlap between LUTS associated with BPH and symptoms associated with CP/CPPS. Although CP/CPPS was traditionally believed to be related to prostatic inflammation or infection, current thinking suggests that although infection/inflammation could be an initiating factor, other variables such as neurogenic, endocrine, immunologic, and psychological factors likely play a role.

Further research into male LUTS and CP/CPPS is vital. With an aging population, the prevalence of bothersome LUTS will increase with a resulting decrease in QOL. At present, diagnosis and assessment of disease severity for patients suffering from benign prostate disease are aided not only through physical exam, but also through the use of numerous validated questionnaires, many of which focus on specific prostate conditions (e.g., BPH/LUTS, incontinence, chronic prostatitis, etc.). Some important issues to consider in assessing the disease phenotype of patients with benign prostate disease are described as follows:

Important Phenotyping Criteria for Patients with Benign Prostate Disease

- Age—BPH is a chronic progressive condition that worsens with age. Longitudinal population studies such as the Olmstead County Study of Urinary Symptoms and Health Status among Men have shown an increase in the incidence of moderate or severe urinary symptoms from 13 percent in the 5th to 28 percent in the 8th decade of life.[1] Age, normal androgenic function, and a positive family history are all risk factors for BPH. Other possible risk factors include race, geographic location,

cigarette smoking, and male pattern baldness. Most patients have pathologic BPH/LUTS by age 60, although only 51 percent of these patients will cite impairment of daily activities as compared to 28 percent of men without BPH. Of these 51 percent of patients, 17 percent complain of this impairment continuously. In other words, roughly 20 percent of patients warrant some form of intervention.

- Symptoms (storage versus voiding) Profiles—LUTS caused by BPH may include frequency, urgency, hesitancy, nocturia (i.e., excessive frequency of urination at night-time), a sensation of incomplete emptying, a weak urinary stream, and post-void dribbling. Our challenge is to develop both diagnostic and therapeutic algorithms that are more comprehensive and encompass different profiles of male LUTS. Today, it is more appropriate to identify male LUTS in terms of storage versus voiding symptoms. Specifically, overactive bladder (OAB) is a syndrome characterized by urinary urgency, with or without urgency urinary incontinence, and usually with frequency and nocturia. These symptoms, therefore, represent a subset of LUTS. However, the concomitant existence of OAB symptoms and prostatic conditions (e.g., benign enlargement of the prostate and bladder outlet obstruction) in men adds complexity to the diagnosis and appropriate treatment. Men with OAB symptoms are more often prescribed pharmacotherapies that target the prostate (e.g., alpha-receptor antagonists, 5-alpha-reductase inhibitors) rather than the bladder (e.g., antimuscarinics).

- Prostate Size—An enlarged prostate is the hallmark of what urologists typically consider BPH. Large, placebo-controlled pharmacological studies have shown that the natural history of the disease can be altered and the incidence of BPH progression reduced by shrinking the prostate with 5-alpha-reductase inhibition.[2,3] Though an enlarged prostate is not always associated with LUTS, across populations prostate volume has been shown to be a consistent marker for future disease progression.

- Inflammation—Tissue specimens from men with LUTS and/or BPH have chronic inflammatory infiltrates in more than 50 percent of the cases. There is growing interest in the area of inflammation in the prostate, both for BPH and prostate carcinogenesis. Studies have shown that patients with chronic inflammatory infiltrates had a higher rate of symptom progression, acute urinary retention, and need for prostate surgery as compared to those without such infiltrates.[4] These observations suggest a greater role for chronic inflammation in the natural history of BPH than previously assumed.

- Cellular Pathology—Histological BPH (i.e., BPH characterized by a non-malignant proliferation of prostate cells that may or may not be associated with symptoms) is composed of a mixture of ratios of glandular epithelial and stromal tissue, the latter being further divided into smooth muscle and connective tissue. The relative proportion of glandular epithelial to stromal tissue changes from young adulthood to older age, and also is different between individuals of the same age.[5] To enhance efficacy, avoid treatment failures, and improve cost effectiveness, further research into patient symptom phenotypes and specific therapies for LUTS, BPH, and CP/CPPS should be conducted. These should take into consideration pathological criteria, including the relative ratios of glandular epithelial and stromal components.

- Imaging Results—Currently, modalities used to image the prostate include ultrasound, magnetic resonance, and computerized axial tomography imaging. These are all currently available clinical techniques, and various advancements have refined their ability to image more accurately and extract both structural and functional information. The area of prostate imaging is currently fertile ground for innovation and new technologies, such as positron emission tomography, new magnetic resonance imaging and ultrasound imaging, magnetic resonance spectroscopy, and the refinement of these technologies with computer-generated 3-D and 4-D perspectives. Finally, the greatest impact these technologies may have is in imaging-assisted therapeutics. Many of the new technologies, such as injection therapies for the prostate, cryotherapy, high intensity ultrasound, as well as robot-assisted procedures, rely on imaging modalities like ultrasound. The evolution of these technologies will have great impact not only in the patient diagnosis, but also in improvement of therapies.

- Comorbid Conditions—LUTS and sexual dysfunction (e.g., ED, ejaculatory dysfunction, etc.) are highly prevalent comorbid conditions in men. The strong associations between LUTS and sexual dysfunction are independent of age and other comorbidities, such as heart disease and diabetes.[6] There is published evidence linking disorders of the prostate (and bladder) with LUTS and sexual dysfunction. However, metabolic, cardiovascular, and endocrine disorders also are likely contributors. Studies of cellular alterations associated with metabolic syndrome and cardiovascular disease are critical to our understanding of the links between LUTS and ED. Readily measured endocrine, metabolic, and cardiovascular parameters may give clinicians clues to possible changes in the cellular mechanisms linked to ED and LUTS. For example, metabolic syndrome is characterized by glucose intolerance (i.e., type II diabetes), elevated fasting plasma glucose, insulin resistance, central obesity, dyslipidemia, and hypertension. Results from the Baltimore Longitudinal Study of Aging demonstrated that men with elevated fasting glucose were three times as likely to have enlarged prostates than were men with normal fasting glucose levels, and men with diabetes were more than twice as likely to have enlarged prostates as men without diabetes. Studies in animal models suggest that the link between the metabolic syndrome and ED and LUTS may include three cellular mechanisms: NO/cGMP signaling, autonomic activity, and Rho-kinase activation. Although difficult to confirm animal findings in humans, studies suggest that identification of abnormalities in fasting blood glucose levels, serum lipid profiles, and blood pressure may help identify factors contributing to LUTS and ED. Also, changes in testosterone levels may contribute to metabolic and cardiovascular changes that may promote the development of LUTS and ED. Consideration of these complex relationships may broaden our approach to managing male pelvic health.

Research Priorities and Recommendations

Age

- Improve our understanding of the relationship between age and other phenotypic criteria, such as symptom profiles, pathology, inflammation, prostate size, biomarker profiles, and imaging results.

Symptoms

- Promote development of improved and comprehensive tools for assessing patient symptom profiles, including storage, voiding, and post-micturition symptoms.
- Study the impact of different symptom constellations on QOL.

Prostate Size

- Improve our understanding of the relationship between prostate size and other phenotypic criteria, such as symptom profiles, pathology, inflammation, biomarker profiles, and imaging results.

Inflammation

- Address the nature of the inflammatory infiltrates (e.g., cell types, etc) present in various benign prostate diseases.
- Identify additional pathological or symptomatic findings associated with the presence of these infiltrates.
- Identify potential serum or other body fluid markers that correlate with the presence of immunological infiltrates.
- Identify therapeutic avenues directed at general or specific inflammatory processes.

Cellular Pathology

- Continue research efforts for phenotype-specific therapies for LUTS, BPH, and CP/CPPS based on respective pathological criteria. This is an important priority for enhancing efficacy, avoiding treatment failures, and improving cost effectiveness.

Imaging Methodologies

- Refine operator independent measurement methodology for ultrasound and nuclear magnetic resonance imaging, as well as improve our ability to image different prostate areas.
- Test the combining of technologies, such as contrast enhanced scanning and spectroscopy, in synergizing effectiveness in imaging the prostate.

Co-Morbid Conditions

- Study the relationships between LUTS/BPH and sexual dysfunction (e.g., ED), as well as other male pelvic disorders.
- Study the relationship between the various manifestations of metabolic syndrome and LUTS/BPH.
- Develop new therapeutic strategies developed from a better understanding of co-morbid relationships.
- Create preventive strategies aimed at underlying common pathophysiologies, such as endothelial dysfunction in aging men.
- Perform a detailed assessment of testosterone levels, especially in older men, to assess urologic and non-urologic conditions underlying LUTS and ED.

General Recommendation

- Study the causes of male LUTS and its association with other conditions based on suggestions from recent scientific observations. Such research may well lead to the definition of specific "phenotypes" of patients and a better definition of disease (e.g., size versus morphological characteristics and their relative importance in producing symptoms, obstructive versus irritative symptoms relative to prostate morphology and size, and CP/CPPS patient phenotypes relative to urologic symptom profiles). This may promote targeted therapeutic strategies, either with interventions currently available, or new strategies that might be discovered as a result of a better understanding of the etiology of the various phenotypes.

References:

1. Chute CG, Panser LA, Girman CJ, et al. The prevalence of prostatism: a population-based survey of urinary symptoms. *Journal of Urology* 1993;150(1):85–89.

2. McConnell JD, Bruskewitz R, Walsh P, et al. The effect of finasteride on the risk of acute urinary retention and the need for surgical treatment among men with benign prostatic hyperplasia. Finasteride Long-Term Efficacy and Safety Study Group. *The New England Journal of Medicine* 1998;338(9):557–563.

3. McConnell JD, Roehrborn CG, Bautista OM, et al. The long-term effect of doxazosin, finasteride, and combination therapy on the clinical progression of benign prostatic hyperplasia. *The New England Journal of Medicine* 2003;349(25):2387–2398.

4. Roehrborn CG, Lukkarinen O, Mark S, Siami P, Ramsdell J, Zinner N. Long-term sustained improvement in symptoms of benign prostatic hyperplasia with the dual 5-alpha-reductase inhibitor dutasteride: results of 4-year studies. *BJU International* 2005;96(4):572–577.

5. Shapiro E, Becich MJ, Hartanto V, Lepor H. The relative proportion of stromal and epithelial hyperplasia is related to the development of symptomatic benign prostate hyperplasia. *Journal of Urology* 1992;147(5):1293–1297.

6. Rosen R, Altwein J, Boyle P, et al. Lower urinary tract symptoms and male sexual dysfunction: the multinational survey of the aging male (MSAM-7). *European Urology* 2003;44(6):637–649.

Our growing realization of the complexity of benign prostate disease raises the question of whether currently available questionnaire instruments used to objectively measure symptom frequency and severity, as well as disease outcomes following treatment, are too narrow for research studies, and perhaps even clinical practice.

The symptoms attributed to benign prostate pathology and their relationship with other disorders, such as ED, are now measured by a host of different instruments. One of the most widely used instruments is the seven-item American Urological Association (AUA) Symptom Index (AUASI). The AUASI was developed with a focus on symptoms thought attributable to prostate dysfunction and secondary changes in the bladder, also thought ultimately attributable to the prostate.[1] The International Prostate Symptom Score (IPSS) questionnaire incorporates the AUASI and adds a separately scored global "bother" question. A separate Symptom Problem Index and a BPH Impact Index focus on the bother of individual symptoms and the impact of the global collection of symptoms on different aspects of health status.[2] A newer questionnaire, the ICSmaleSF, has 13 items scored in a separate voiding scale (five items), an incontinence scale (six items), and separate items on frequency and nocturia.[3] The NIH-Chronic Pain Symptom Index (NIH-CPSI) was developed to quantify symptoms possibly related to CP/CPPS.[4] Nine items are scored in three scales: pain (four items), urinary symptoms (two items), and impact of symptoms/QOL (three items). Neither the IPSS nor the ICSmaleSF include questions about pain, which is traditionally thought to be the distinguishing symptom of CP/CPPS.

The number and variation of the currently accepted instruments, as well as our changing views of disease etiology, suggest it is time to re-evaluate our assessment of symptom frequency and severity and the relationship between organ-specific pathology and symptoms. Attempting to achieve consensus on an appropriate "core" of symptoms to measure and the relevant instruments to measure them is fundamental to advancing clinical research in male lower urinary tract dysfunction resulting from benign disease of the prostate.

- Convene a multidisciplinary working group to develop a specific research agenda for symptom and health status measurement related to male (or perhaps both male and female) lower urinary tract dysfunction. Investigators interested in the broad spectrum of underlying conditions, the architects of prominent instruments, as well as thought leaders from professional societies and government organizations, should be invited. Areas of uncertainty and disputes should be clarified by prospective studies prioritized by the group.

Examples of specific key questions to be addressed in future efforts may include, but would not be limited to:

- Which symptoms belong to which "domains" (e.g., should urge incontinence be scaled along with urgency and other voiding symptoms)?
- Which symptoms and scales are most strongly related to disease-specific and overall health status?
- Which scales should be included as a minimum "core package" in future clinical studies involving the urinary tract, regardless of the disease focus?
- What is the current state of understanding of how various pathologic processes cause symptoms and what studies would clarify those relationships?
- Should the focus of core symptom questionnaires move primarily from frequency or severity to bother or impact?
- How should response to treatment be assessed and considered in validating core symptom scales (given that a poor response may reflect an unresponsive questionnaire or simply a weak treatment effect)?
- How should different scales addressing similar domains be compared in prospective studies and what would constitute evidence that one scale is "better" than another?
- How should respondent burden and practicality be assessed and considered in developing a core set of scales?
- How should "minimal perceptible differences" be defined for core symptom questionnaires to determine what levels of change are clinically important?

References:

1. Barry MJ, Fowler FJ, Jr., O'Leary MP, et al. The American Urological Association symptom index for benign prostatic hyperplasia. The Measurement Committee of the American Urological Association. *Journal of Urology* 1992;148(5):1549–1557.

2. Barry MJ, Fowler FJ, Jr., O'Leary MP, Bruskewitz RC, Holtgrewe HL, Mebust WK. Measuring disease-specific health status in men with benign prostatic hyperplasia. Measurement Committee of The American Urological Association. *Medical Care* 1995;33(4 Suppl):AS145–AS155.

3. Donovan JL, Peters TJ, Abrams P, Brookes ST, de aa Rosette JJ, Schafer W. Scoring the short form ICSmaleSF questionnaire. International Continence Society. *Journal of Urology* 2000;164(6):1948–1955.

4. Litwin MS, McNaughton-Collins M, Fowler FJ, Jr., et al. The National Institutes of Health chronic prostatitis symptom index: development and validation of a new outcome measure. Chronic Prostatitis Collaborative Research Network. *Journal of Urology* 1999;162(2):369–375.

30. Issues in Clinical Trial Design

General Trial Design Issues

Clinical trials of medical treatments seek to compare the effect of treatments on targeted outcomes, usually for both therapeutic benefits and unintended harm, in a group of appropriate patients. A potentially active treatment (e.g., medication, device, surgery) is often compared against a placebo or sham procedure. The "gold standard" for parallel treatment comparisons involves random allocation of subjects to treatment, with the goal of attempting to balance the distribution of prognostic factors between the groups to be compared, thus isolating the effect of the treatments being compared.

In recent years, the Consolidated Standards of Reporting Trials (CONSORT) group has published criteria for improving the quality of reporting of parallel-group randomized trials.[1] These criteria have recently been extended to cover the better reporting of harms in randomized trials, better reporting of cluster randomized trials, and better reporting of non-inferiority and equivalence trials.[2,3] Inevitably, higher standards for reporting trials should lead to more thoughtful design of trials.

Traditional clinical "efficacy" trials generally test interventions in settings and populations carefully selected so the treatment can show a maximum effect. However, positive results from such trials may not be "generalizable" to actual practice "in the trenches." Practical or "effectiveness" trials are conducted in real practice settings with broader groups of patients, and may generate results that are more generalizable to the "typical patient" and therefore, more readily translated into practice. However, effects can be heterogeneous using such large groups and thus, they may miss therapeutic (or harmful) effects in more narrowly defined subsets of patients.

A key decision in the design of a clinical trial is the selection of appropriate outcome measures for a best assessment of therapy effectiveness. Decisions need to include not only which outcome measures to use, but also how many there should be, that are considered "primary," and how should the minimum clinically important differences in the primary outcomes be defined for sample size calculations.

Research Priorities and Recommendations

- Establish a benign prostate disease clinical trials network to develop multiple trial strategies simultaneously, rather than the inefficient, one-at-a-time clinical trial design and execution system.
- Promote collaborations with the AUA for systematic literature reviews for BPH. The AUA's guidelines program conducts systematic literature reviews of clinical trials in prostate diseases and this review is currently being updated for BPH. This effort may be an efficient way to translate research priorities defined by the guideline effort into new high-priority trials.

Specific Trial Design Issues

Many important questions in the diagnosis and treatment of benign prostate disorders, such as male LUTS and clinical BPH (i.e., BPH involving symptoms), have been addressed over the past 15 years using various traditional trial designs. Each of these offer unique advantages and disadvantages.[4] Descriptions of some of these designs, as well as select, relevant companion resources are listed below:

- Cross-sectional population-based studies offer a snapshot of the distribution of signs, symptoms, and other investigated parameters across a chosen population stratified usually by factors such as gender, age, and other parameters.

- Longitudinal population-based studies can provide greater informational value, as the same population is followed over time. This allows a study of the natural history of the signs, symptoms, and other parameters of disease. Tremendous insights have been gained from such studies. For example, the Olmsted County Study of Urinary Symptoms in Men has contributed more than 100 scientific articles to our knowledge base.[5,6,7,8] The Boston Area Community Health Survey is an NIH-sponsored longitudinal study in a very well-characterized and stratified population of men and women in the Boston area and is likely to yield yet new insights into the epidemiology and natural history of female and male LUTS.[9,10,11,12]

- Disease registries are unique vehicles for the study of a condition and/or the impact of interventions on conditions. Registries allow for a less restricted interaction between health care providers and patients compared to controlled trials, and thus facilitate studies of treatments, symptom severity, etc. The ongoing and continued use of disease-specific registries, perhaps as web-based endeavors, are encouraged as a vehicle to accumulate knowledge about differences in the delivery of health care, practice patterns, and the treatment of benign prostate disease.

- A vast majority of clinical studies in the field are randomized controlled clinical trials (RCTs), usually implying a parallel group design, multicenter setting, double or at least single blinding, and controlled study of the efficacy and safety of one or more interventions. Although the list of RCTs is long and exhaustive, there are several specific areas of interest that remain poorly understood and/or under researched, such as the role of the placebo.

  – Placebo effect and role of placebo lead-in—There is a tremendous placebo effect noted in nearly all RCTs in male LUTS for nearly all assessed parameters. It is understood that this effect is partially a unilateral regression to the mean effect induced by the inclusion and exclusion criteria, though effects due simply to interactions with the health care providers in a clinical setting or other "placebo" related effect are possible contributors. Many trials have a placebo lead-in period, but others do not. Some mandate rescreening after the placebo lead-in, while others do not. These differences lead to different ultimate outcomes in terms of the magnitude of the effect of the studied intervention. A better understanding of the role, effect, and limitations exerted by the use or non-use of the placebo lead-in would be of significant interest to the field and regulatory authorities. One advantage would be to establish a more level playing field for the different drugs and interventions. For example, there is no comparable "sham lead-in" for surgical trials and, therefore, the interventions are credited for the full observed effect (i.e., placebo plus actual benefit).

  – Placebo or active compound withdrawal studies—The effect of drug withdrawal is very little on the signs and symptoms of benign prostate disease. There is only one study that formally reports on the effect of combination therapy and the symptomatic consequences of a placebo-controlled withdrawal of one of the two drugs.[13]

    A detailed study of the role of the placebo lead-in and its impact on ultimate outcomes, as well as detailed studies of placebo-controlled drug withdrawals over time would add significantly to our understanding of the best policies in medical therapies for benign prostate disease such as male LUTS.

- To the extent it is possible and important to define phenotypes of patients based on a variety of parameters (see section on phenotyping), phenotype-driven trials are an important future tool to assess the clinical validity of such definitions and assignments. One might also consider such efforts as proof-of-concept trials. For example, if a phytotherapeutic compound claims to act as an anti-inflammatory (or antiphlogistic) agent, it should follow that such an agent has its best efficacy in patients who in fact have an inflammatory component to their condition. The appropriate way of testing such a hypothesis would be to select men based on biopsy findings of inflammatory infiltrates and treat them with such a compound. An ideal trial design also would call for a placebo or other control. A further refinement would be to enroll all patients but stratify by baseline presence or absence of inflammation and maintain blinding to study the investigator and patients, and, therefore, analyze the response to placebo versus active compound in men with and without inflammatory infiltrates. Further phenotype-driven trials, with and without enrollment stratified by phenotype, and preferentially with a control arm, are a priority.

- From a public health point of view, dealing effectively with a condition means to prevent the condition. In the area of male LUTS (e.g., clinical BPH), only secondary prevention of outcomes of the condition has been contemplated and studied. Secondary prevention of complications and outcomes, such as acute urinary retention and need for prostate-related surgery, has been shown to be preventable in about 50 percent of cases by the long-term use of 5-alpha-reductase inhibitors (e.g., finasteride and dutasteride).[14,15,16] Primary prevention of the condition has, to our knowledge, not been attempted. The search for and study of primary prevention for benign prostate disease, such as male LUTS, is an important priority for the future.

Research Priorities and Recommendations

- Foster collaboration with existing, longitudinal population-based studies to assist investigators in answering relevant questions.
- Encourage the continued and ongoing use of disease-specific registries, perhaps as web-based endeavors, as a vehicle to accumulate knowledge about differences in the delivery of health care, practice patterns, and the treatment of male LUTS (e.g., clinical BPH) unrestricted by a controlled clinical trial setting.
- Consider how certain clinical questions would benefit from a systematic use of non-randomized observation trials, while in other cases, preference trials would aid our understanding of the impact of interventions on the condition.
- Give priority to trials of strategies (e.g., clinical practice or real life practice trials) and further phenotype-driven trials, with and without

enrollment stratified by phenotype and preferentially with a control arm.
- Recognize that the search for and study of primary prevention for BPH/LUTS is an important priority in the future.

The following should be promoted:

- The sharing of trial protocols, data, and statistical code with other investigators to promote transparent, reproducible, and trustworthy research.
- The dissemination of trial results through novel means, including professional guidelines and patient decision aids.

Recommendations for the Development of a Clinical Trial Infrastructure

- Develop a collaborative network to standardize treatment assessment. The creation of a LUTS Treatment Collaborative Network (LTCN) would allow the critical aggregation of thought leaders. By the rapid adoption and completion of trials, the network could increase throughput and help to identify promising concepts in treatment and prevention of male LUTS.
- Enhance collaboration among Federal agencies. There is great risk that one Federal agency may pursue goals that are not recognized as critical by other agencies.
- Develop a web-based network of community treated patients (i.e., a benign prostate disease treatment registry). Placebo-controlled, double-masked trials remain the gold standard in assessing drug impact in male LUTS treatment. However, in some circumstances patient treatment registries could be used as vehicles for the study of a condition and/or the impact of interventions on the conditions. This may allow for a less restricted interaction between health care providers and patients compared to controlled trials, and thus facilitate the study of the natural evolution of treatment cascades, symptom severity threshold triggering therapeutic interactions, etc.

References:

1. Moher D, Schulz KF, Altman D. The CONSORT statement: revised recommendations for improving the quality of reports of parallel-group randomized trials. *JAMA: The Journal of the American Medical Association* 2001;285(15):1987–1991.

2. Ioannidis JP, Evans SJ, Gotzsche PC, et al. Better reporting of harms in randomized trials: an extension of the CONSORT statement. *Annals of Internal Medicine* 2004;141(10):781–788.

References (continued):

3. Campbell MK, Elbourne DR, Altman DG. CONSORT statement: extension to cluster randomised trials. *British Medical Journal (Clinical research ed)* 2004;328(7441):702–708.

4. Roehrborn C, McConnell JD. Etiology, pathophysiology, epidemiology and natural history of benign prostatic hyperplasia. In: Walsh PC, Retik AB, Vaughan ED, Jr., Wein AJ, Kavoussi LR, Novick AC, et al. (eds.). *Campbell's Urology.* 8th ed. Philadelphia, PA: WB Saunders Co.: 2002, pp. 1297–1336.

5. Chute CG, Panser LA, Girman CJ, et al. The prevalence of prostatism: a population-based survey of urinary symptoms. *Journal of Urology* 1993;150(1):85–89.

6. Roberts RO, Rhodes T, Panser LA, et al. Natural history of prostatism: worry and embarrassment from urinary symptoms and health care-seeking behavior. *Urology* 1994;43(5):621–628.

7. Guess HA, Jacobsen SJ, Girman CJ, et al. The role of community-based longitudinal studies in evaluating treatment effects. Example: benign prostatic hyperplasia. *Medical Care* 1995;33(4 Suppl):AS26–AS35.

8. Rhodes T, Girman CJ, Jacobsen SJ, Guess HA, Oesterling JE, Lieber MM. Longitudinal measures of prostate volume in a community-based sample: 3.5 year followup in the Olmsted County Study of health status and urinary symptoms among men. *Journal of Urology* 1995;153:301A abstract 291.

9. Kupelian V, Wei JT, O'Leary MP, et al. Prevalence of lower urinary tract symptoms and effect on quality of life in a racially and ethnically diverse random sample: the Boston Area Community Health (BACH) Survey. *Archives of Internal Medicine* 2006;166(21):2381–2387.

10. Link CL, Lutfey KE, Steers WD, McKinlay JB. Is abuse causally related to urologic symptoms? Results from the Boston Area Community Health (BACH) Survey. *European Urology* 2007;52(2):397–406.

11. McKinlay JB, Link CL. Measuring the urologic iceberg: design and implementation of the Boston Area Community Health (BACH) Survey. *European Urology* 2007;52(2):389–396.

12. Robertson C, Link CL, Onel E, et al. The impact of lower urinary tract symptoms and comorbidities on quality of life: the BACH and UREPIK studies. *BJU International* 2007;99(2):347–354.

13. Barkin J, Guimaraes M, Jacobi G, Pushkar D, Taylor S, Vierssen Trip OB. Alpha-blocker therapy can be withdrawn in the majority of men following initial combination therapy with the dual 5-alpha-reductase inhibitor dutasteride. *European Urology* 2003;44(4):461–466.

14. McConnell JD, Bruskewitz R, Walsh P, et al. The effect of finasteride on the risk of acute urinary retention and the need for surgical treatment among men with benign prostatic hyperplasia. Finasteride Long-Term Efficacy and Safety Study Group. *The New England Journal of Medicine* 1998;338(9):557–563.

15. Roehrborn CG, Boyle P, Nickel JC, Hoefner K, Andriole G. Efficacy and safety of a dual inhibitor of 5-alpha-reductase types 1 and 2 (dutasteride) in men with benign prostatic hyperplasia. *Urology* 2002;60(3):434–441.

16. Roehrborn CG, Lukkarinen O, Mark S, Siami P, Ramsdell J, Zinner N. Long-term sustained improvement in symptoms of benign prostatic hyperplasia with the dual 5-alpha-reductase inhibitor dutasteride: results of 4-year studies. *BJU International* 2005;96(4):572–577.

31. Specific Clinical Trial Study Concepts: Drug Therapy

Alpha-Blocker Therapy

There is an extensive database of trials using all four of the currently available alpha-adrenergic receptor blockers (i.e., "alpha-blockers") for the treatment of BPH/LUTS: alfuzosin, doxazosin, tamsulosin, and terazosin. Although the majority of these trials are short- to intermediate-term (< 12 weeks in duration) and purely standard efficacy and safety trials, there are exceptions: The Veterans Affairs Cooperative Study and the Prospective European Doxazosin and Combination Therapy Study are 12-month long trials with terazosin and doxazosin,[1,2] the Alfuzosin Long-Term Efficacy and Safety Study is a 2-year progression trial with alfuzosin,[3] and Medical Therapy of Prostatic Symptoms is a 5-year progression trial including doxazosin.[4] It is generally accepted that all alpha-blockers are of equal efficacy, but have a slightly different side-effect profile. It has become clear that the precise mechanism of action of alpha-blockers is not as simple as previously proposed (i.e., relaxation of smooth muscle in bladder neck and prostate).

Research Priorities and Recommendations

*   Derive a better understanding of the mechanism(s) of action of alpha-blockers in men with LUTS.
*   Develop trials to further understand differences in terms of adverse events and side effects for the different alpha-blockers.
*   Assess the differential effect of alpha-blockers on voiding versus storage symptoms.
*   Study the efficacy of alpha-blockers in intermittent versus continuous treatment (i.e., in terms of waxing and waning of symptoms).
*   Assess the usefulness of alpha-blockers in the treatment of men with CP/CPPS.

5-alpha-reductase Inhibitors

The 5-alpha-reductase inhibitors dutasteride and finasteride have demonstrated long-term efficacy and safety in 1- to 5-year long clinical trials.[5,6,7] The mechanism of action has been well established as a hormonal withdrawal-induced atrophy of the glandular epithelial component of the prostate tissue. This class of drugs also may suppress the expression of vascular endothelial growth factor in the suburethral glandular tissue and, therefore, may affect prostate-related bleeding, hematospermia (i.e., the presence of blood in semen), and/or perioperative bleeding surrounding transurethral procedures. A recent study, however, suggested no effect at least in regards to the latter.[8]

Research Priorities and Recommendations

- Address the differential effect of these drugs on serum prostate specific antigen (PSA) in men with LUTS only versus men with LUTS and undiagnosed prostate cancer.
- Assess the differential effects of different 5-alpha-reductase inhibitor classes in LUTS.
- Assess the usefulness of 5-alpha-reductase inhibitors in the treatment of men with CP/CPPS.

Antimuscarinic Drugs

Antimuscarinic drugs, which block bladder muscarinic acetylcholine receptors thus inhibiting contraction, have been thought to be contraindicated in men with LUTS and BPH out of fear of inducing problems with urinary retention. Recent evidence from short- to intermediate-term studies suggests that this risk may have been overestimated. There is ample room for research in the area of antimuscarinics in men with LUTS, OAB, and BPH.

Research Priorities and Recommendations

- Establish the long-term safety of antimuscarinic drugs.
- Assess the efficacy and safety of antimuscarinic drugs in populations stratified by prostate size, serum PSA, age, peak flow rate, and post-void residual.
- Assess combination therapy in phenotype-stratified populations.
- Study muscarinic receptors in the prostate and their role in male LUTS.

PDE-5 Inhibitors

The newest class of drugs to be studied in male LUTS is the PDE-5 inhibitors. Although clearly representing the standard of care in the management of ED, the three drugs in the class—sildenafil citrate, tadalefil, and vardenafil—all have been shown to improve LUTS in men when using standardized instruments to measure symptom severity, frequency, bother, and quality of life (QOL).[9,10] Of interest, neither one of the drugs appears to influence other measures, such as post-void residual (PVR) or maximum urinary flow rate.

Research Priorities and Recommendations

- Support studies of mechanism(s) of PDE-5 inhibitor action.
- Assess the differential response regarding voiding versus storage symptoms for PDE-5 inhibitor therapy.
- Assess the urodynamic effect in models and/or full-scale urodynamic trials.
- Study the safety and efficacy in long-term daily administration for PDE-5 inhibitor therapy.
- Assess the role of potential combination therapies including PDE-5 inhibitors.

Anti-Inflammatory Agents

With the exception of very small, short, and poorly or not at all controlled studies, there has been virtually no clinical trials studying the potential use of anti-inflammatory agents in men with LUTS. There is abundant opportunity for basic, translational, and clinical research addressing the role of inflammation and anti-inflammatory agents in the management of men with benign prostate disease.

Research Priorities and Recommendations

- Explore further characterization of inflammatory infiltrates (e.g., cell types, tissue/body fluid/serum markers, epidemiological data on frequency and severity of infiltrates, etc.).
- Verify efficacy and safety of anti-inflammatory agents for benign prostate disease in men stratified by presence versus absence of inflammation.

With four to five classes of drugs available as potential treatments, the testing of various combinations of these drugs in terms of enhanced efficacy and better safety is a significant research priority. Table 1 illustrates key drug classes, their presumed mechanisms of action, their positive attributes, and their adverse event spectrum.

- Test a variety of combinations other than the already established combination of alpha-blocker with 5-reductase-inhibitors in phenotype-stratified patient populations.
- Assess combination therapy employing neuromodulatory drugs for benign prostate disease.
- Assess combination therapy employing immunomodulatory agents for CP/CPPS.

Table 1 Characteristics of various drug therapies.

Class	Presumed Mechanism	Effect	Adverse Effects
α-blocker	Smooth muscle relaxation Effects in spinal cord (?) Central effects (?)	Symptom ▼▼ Flow rate ▲ Progression (.)	Dizziness Hypotension Ejaculation ▼
5 ARI	Conversion of T to DHT Atropy/apoptosis Volume shrinkage	Symptom ▼ Flow rate ▲ Progress ▼▼▼	Erection ▼ Libido ▼ Ejaculation ▼
Antimuscarinic	Anticholinergic bladder effect	Symptom ▼▼ Flow rate (. to ▼) Progression (.)	Dry mouth
PDE-5 inhibitor	Muscle relaxation analogous to corpora cavernosa (?)	Symptom ▼▼ Flow rate (.) Progression (?)	Erection ▲▲▲ Ejaculation ▲

References:

1. Lepor H, Williford WO, Barry MJ, et al. The efficacy of terazosin, finasteride, or both in benign prostatic hyperplasia. Veterans Affairs Cooperative Studies Benign Prostatic Hyperplasia Study Group. *The New England Journal of Medicine* 1996;335(8):533–539.

2. Kirby RS, Roehrborn C, Boyle P, et al. Efficacy and tolerability of doxazosin and finasteride, alone or in combination, in treatment of symptomatic benign prostatic hyperplasia: the Prospective European Doxazosin and Combination Therapy (PREDICT) trial. *Urology* 2003;61(1):119–126.

3. McNeill SA, Hargreave TB, Roehrborn CG. Alfuzosin 10 mg once daily in the management of acute urinary retention: results of a double-blind placebo-controlled study. *Urology* 2005;65(1):83–89.

4. McConnell JD, Roehrborn CG, Bautista OM, et al. The long-term effect of doxazosin, finasteride, and combination therapy on the clinical progression of benign prostatic hyperplasia. *The New England Journal of Medicine* 2003;349(25):2387–2398.

5. McConnell JD, Bruskewitz R, Walsh P, et al. The effect of finasteride on the risk of acute urinary retention and the need for surgical treatment among men with benign prostatic hyperplasia. Finasteride Long-Term Efficacy and Safety Study Group. *The New England Journal of Medicine* 1998;338(9):557–563.

6. Roehrborn CG, Lukkarinen O, Mark S, Siami P, Ramsdell J, Zinner N. Long-term sustained improvement in symptoms of benign prostatic hyperplasia with the dual 5-alpha-reductase inhibitor dutasteride: results of 4-year studies. *BJU International* 2005;96(4):572–577.

7. McConnell JD, Roehrborn CG, Bautista OM, et al. The long-term effect of doxazosin, finasteride, and combination therapy on the clinical progression of benign prostatic hyperplasia. *The New England Journal of Medicine* 2003;349(25):2387–2398.

8. Hahn RG, Fagerstrom T, Tammela TL, et al. Blood loss and postoperative complications associated with transurethral resection of the prostate after pretreatment with dutasteride. *BJU International* 2007;99(3):587–594.

9. McVary KT, Monnig W, Camps JL, Jr., Young JM, Tseng LJ, van den EG. Sildenafil citrate improves erectile function and urinary symptoms in men with erectile dysfunction and lower urinary tract symptoms associated with benign prostatic hyperplasia: a randomized, double-blind trial. *Journal of Urology* 2007;177(3):1071–1077.

10. McVary KT, Roehrborn CG, Kaminetsky JC, et al. Tadalafil relieves lower urinary tract symptoms secondary to benign prostatic hyperplasia. *Journal of Urology* 2007;177(4):1401–1407.

Phytotherapeutic agents (i.e., agents derived from extracts from plants or other natural sources) are commonly prescribed in Europe for LUTS. In the United States, 30 to 90 percent of patients seen by urologists for BPH/LUTS may be taking them over the counter. The U.S. market for dietary supplements to treat LUTS or just "to keep the prostate healthy" is around $1.5 billion in sales per year, with U.S. supplement sales now totaling more than $8 billion. Phytotherapeutic agents are herbal preparations made by various extraction processes to obtain a complex mixture of ingredient plant materials. Table 1 outlines some of the numerous components of plant extracts.

Table 1. Components of Herbal Preparations for BPH

Phytosterols (β-sitosterol, campesterol, stigmasterol, Δ⁷-sterols, Δ⁵-sterols)
Lupenone
Lupeol
Terpenoids
Fatty acids (free, long-chain, short-chain)
Lectins
Plant oils
Polysaccharides
Flavonoids
Phytoestrogens (coumestrol, genistein)
Phenols

After a long period of minimal scrutiny, in June 2007, the U.S. Food and Drug Administration (FDA) announced a stricter policy for the regulation of dietary supplements that would require manufacturers to evaluate "the identity, purity, quality, strength, and composition of dietary supplements."

More lenient restrictions have made phytotherapeutic agents more available to consumers since 1994, but in addition to their uncertain value for restoring health, recent reports suggest a number of harmful effects. Despite these reports, the general public still believes that these "natural" products carry no toxicity.

Unlike standard pharmaceutical products, which undergo extensive testing, phytotherapies have never been tested for bioavailability. There are no data available about absorption or excretion of any of the phytotherapeutic products currently being sold over the counter. These studies should be undertaken once the pharmacological active components are identified.

Central to the understanding of the field of phytotherapy is determining the mechanism of action. Many different mechanisms of action have been proposed for the phytotherapies used for BPH/LUTS (Table 2). These products are believed to act as anti-inflammatory agents acting on prostaglandin synthesis and metabolism, as anti-androgenic agents through their effect on 5-alpha-reductase activity in the nuclear membrane, and as modulators of various growth factors.[1,2]

Table 2. Suggested Mechanisms of Action of Plant Extracts

Inhibition of 5-α reductase I and II
Overall anti-inflammatory effect
Anti-edema effect
Overall interference with prostaglandin metabolism
Inhibition of phospholipase A2 and 5-lipoxygenase enzymes
Blockage of the release of arachidonic acid
Inhibition of androgen and estrogen receptors
Action on α-adrenergic receptors
Overall anti-estrogenic effect
Overall anti-androgenic effect
Overall suppression of prostate cell metabolism and growth
Induction of cell apoptosis and necrosis
Inhibition of growth factor-induced prostatic cell proliferation
Inhibition of prolactin-induced prostate growth
Decreased sex hormone binding globulin
Free radical scavengers/membrane stabilization
Inhibition of aromatase
Protection and strengthening of detrusor muscle
Overall reduction of prostatic urethral resistance
Alteration of cholesterol metabolism

Research into mechanisms of action for such agents needs to be undertaken in three main areas:

1) Basic *in vitro* laboratory studies to assess the effects in cell culture.
2) *In vivo* animal studies to assess the biochemical, biological, and physiological effects.
3) *In vivo* human studies to assess changes in biomarkers and physiology.

Another important area that has not been addressed is the issue of the interaction between phytotherapies and standard pharmaceutical products. Although the products currently used for BPH/LUTS have not been demonstrated to have any significant drug-drug interactions, this area has not been critically addressed.

Research Priorities and Recommendations

- Support further clinical studies to ascertain whether there is any clinical benefit to phytotherapeutic agents.
- Address the underlying pharmacology of phytotherapeutic agents.
- Establish a pharmacological group to help select the most appropriate products to be studied.

- Identify the composition and function of the constituent substances. Most importantly, determine the understanding of the mechanisms of action through basic *in vitro* experiments as well as *in vivo* studies in animals and proof-of-concept studies in humans.
- Undertake additional randomized, placebo-controlled clinical studies to ascertain the true frequency and magnitude of beneficial effects of relevant phytotherapeutic agents for CP/CPPS.
- Investigate additional complementary medicine studies for CP/CPPS, including: cognitive behavioral modification, dietary modulation, stress reduction, and acupuncture.

References:

1. Bayne CW, Ross M, Donnelly F, Habib FK. The selectivity and specificity of the actions of the lipido-sterolic extract of *Serenoa repens* (Permixon) on the prostate. *Journal of Urology* 2000:164(3 Pt 1):876–881.

2. Buck AC. Is there a scientific basis for the therapeutic effects of *Serenoa repens* in benign prostatic hyperplasia? Mechanisms of action. *Journal of Urology* 2004:172(5 Pt 1):1792–1799.

33. Specific Clinical Trial Study Concepts: Behavioral and Lifestyle Interventions

Many chronic conditions in men and women are effectively treated with self-management programs. For example, self management of diabetes mellitus is a common therapeutic intervention and greatly enhances the efficacy of conventional therapy. It has long been recognized that benign prostate disease, such as BPH/LUTS, has adverse affect on patients' QOL. However, the next logical step, namely to counsel patients regarding their lifestyle activities, has not been widely examined. The concept of self management is reasonably straightforward. Patients are counseled individually or in groups by providers in terms of behavioral changes to positively affect their bothersome symptoms. Studies addressing changes in symptoms and risk factors (e.g., obesity, metabolic syndrome, etc.) through behavioral changes (e.g., fluid avoidance, travel strategies, weight loss, etc.) is a very high research priority.

Treatment of Metabolic Syndrome as a Way of Treating LUTS—Impact of Weight Loss and Exercise

Metabolic syndrome, which is characterized by the presence of a group of metabolic risk factors (e.g., obesity, high blood pressure, poor lipid profile, etc.), has gained recent attention due to its increasing

prevalence in the United States and currently affects more than 47 million people. The presence of metabolic syndrome has been associated with obesity, sedentary lifestyle, and poor cardiovascular fitness. This alarmingly increasing incidence of obesity presents a significant public health concern for the United States and many other developed countries.[1]

Although the exact pathophysiological mechanism is unknown, it is clear that there is an emerging relationship between metabolic syndrome and LUTS. This robust relationship has been unappreciated to date and offers an unexplored means to prevent or even reverse LUTS through behavioral modification therapy directed toward addressing risk factors for metabolic syndrome. Multiple modifiable risk factors have been implicated in increasing the risk of developing metabolic syndrome, including sedentary lifestyle, elevated intake of saturated fats, decreased dietary fiber, and low levels of exercise. Theoretically, if patients could make lifestyle changes to prevent them from developing metabolic syndrome, then these patients may have a decreased risk of developing LUTS as well. The Massachusetts Male Aging Study found that physical exercise served to decrease the risk of developing symptomatic BPH.[2] Another study of 3,743 men between the ages of 40 to 75 years found that physical activity was inversely related to the development of symptomatic LUTS.[3] It remains to be seen whether patients with Metabolic Syndrome who already suffer from LUTS can see an improvement in these symptoms with lifestyle interventions such as exercise.

Research Priorities and Recommendations

* Address intervention studies and assessments of metabolic syndrome and LUTS.
* Investigate topic areas such as:
  – The relationship between obesity and BPH/LUTS.
  – Assess the impact of global lifestyle interventions (e.g., exercise, diet, weight loss) for men at risk for or with an early stage of BPH/LUTS.
  – The influence of arterial hypertension on LUTS/BPH is completely untapped as an avenue for clinical investigation and possible intervention.
  – The interaction between BPH/LUTS and ED also should be examined.
* Study specific hypotheses of how BPH/LUTS is impacted by obesity-related disease and pathophysiologies.
* Organize and promote collaborative efforts between urologists, exercise physiologists, and dietary experts.

Treatment of CP/CPPS through Lifestyle Intervention

Because CP/CPPS has been so difficult to treat with standard pharmaceuticals, numerous lifestyle changes have been suggested as possible interventions. These include avoidance of alcohol and caffeine containing beverages, increased frequency of ejaculation, perineal and pelvic massage therapy, stress reduction, and a vegetarian diet. To date, there is no conclusive evidence that any of these modifications have had significant positive benefit for a majority of the CP/CPPS patients. However, there are some anecdotal and clinical observations that suggest that some patients may benefit from these lifestyle interventions. Concurrent with improved identification and classification of CP/CPPS patients, these modifications should be rigorously tested in appropriate patient cohorts.

Research Priorities and Recommendations

* Encourage innovative studies using behavioral and lifestyle approaches for the treatment of CP/CPPS, such as cognitive behavioral studies and biofeedback, acupuncture, and other alternative interventions.

References:

1. Mokdad AH, Serdula MK, Dietz WH, Bowman BA, Marks JS, Koplan JP. The continuing epidemic of obesity in the United States. *JAMA: The Journal of the American Medical Association* 2000;284(13):1650–1651.

2. Meigs JB, Mohr B, Barry MJ, Collins MM, McKinlay JB. Risk factors for clinical benign prostatic hyperplasia in a community-based population of healthy aging men. *Journal of Clinical Epidemiology* 2001;54(9):935–944.

3. Platz EA, Kawachi I, Rimm EB, et al. Physical activity and benign prostatic hyperplasia. *Archives of Internal Medicine* 1998;158(21):2349–2356.

34. Specific Clinical Trial Study Concepts: Additional Intervention Therapies

Within the last two decades, a plethora of alternative therapies have been developed as options to more standard medical therapies and surgery. Many of these therapies have been introduced as approved alternatives based on short-term efficacy with favorable risk profiles. However, durability or long-term efficacy has persistently remained in controversy due to a lack of convincing large, randomized, prospective, multicenter, comparative studies demonstrating efficacy. Two alternative therapies of growing interest for the treatment of benign prostate disease, specifically BPH/LUTS, are highlighted in the paragraphs that follow.

Injectable Agents

The newest, most novel, and still investigational therapy for treatment of prostate disorders, is injectable pharmacologic intervention. In this class of therapies, an agent is injected into the prostate or other location in the body. The mechanism of action for each agent is varied. One example is Botulinum toxin, which is a neurotoxin and is injected into the prostate via a transurethral or transrectal approach. The efficacy, mechanism of action, and durability are unclear. Despite promise, there is a need for further research to clarify many basic issues.

Thermotherapy as an Alternative to Standard Surgical Interventions

For decades, the only option for BPH treatment was to offer either transurethral resection of the prostate or open prostatectomy to reduce prostatic bladder outlet obstruction. These surgical procedures are associated with well-known QOL complications, such as impotence and incontinence, as well as life-threatening complications. As a result, a plethora of alternative options have developed from medical therapy to minimally invasive therapy to traditional surgical therapy. The options and alternatives are many, and the choice of which procedure is best remains in the domain of the individually treated patient and the treating physician/surgeon.

Minimally invasive thermotherapy has become an option to surgical as well as medical therapy. It offers acceptable efficacy with tolerability and a low threat of adverse events, and expands the treatment population.

Two Current Thermotherapy Technologies and Their Differences

- *Site-Specific Thermotherapy: Transurethral Needle Ablation.* In 1996, the FDA approved the minimally invasive transurethral needle ablation system for the treatment of BPH. Needle electrodes deliver low-level radiofrequency energy precisely into the target tissue. Shields help to protect the urethra from thermal damage. The radiofrequency energy thermally devascularizes and denervates the target tissue, creating necrotic lesions. The radiofrequency energy decreases prostate size by 10–15 percent by heat and dehydration.

- *Non-Site Specific Thermotherapy: Transurethral Microwave Thermotherapy.* The use of microwaves for the treatment of prostate disorders was introduced in the 1990s with transurethral microwave thermotherapy (TUMT). TUMT uses microwave heating to create temperatures greater than 45°C, which is the minimum cytotoxic level of tissue. To create the high interprostatic temperature, water-cooling is often used at the urethra to maintain patient comfort levels. The goal of this therapy is to deinnervate and reduce the size of the prostate to relive symptoms.

Research Priorities and Recommendations

- Continue research of injectable therapies at every level, including basic science studies of the mechanism of action, pharmacologic profile, development of investigative models, as well as clinical trial issues such as modes of delivery and agent placement optimal dosage, safety and efficacy, and patient selection.
- Develop new animal models and artificial models for assessment of new technologies *in vivo*.
- Encourage clinical studies to assess novel new technologies.
- Analyze the baseline parameters for best selection of the patient for surgical intervention.
- Promote technology assessment panels and centers of excellence to allow better clinical studies to validate efficacy and safety of new technologies.
- Encourage comparative prospective long-term studies of currently available technologies, including analysis of technologies with a similar mechanism of action.
- Encourage a cost analysis structure to determine the cost benefit of new technology.
- Analyze and understand the impact of early surgical versus alternative interventions on preventing the outcome of end-stage bladder outlet obstruction.
- Encourage studies that will result in better techniques and training for new technologies by entities that are independent of industry support (e.g., development of virtual simulators).

- Make obesity and lifestyle interventions a priority area for benign prostate disease.
  - Study specific hypotheses of how BPH/LUTS is impacted by obesity, the metabolic syndrome, and related diseases.
  - Organize and promote collaborative efforts between urologists, clinical trialists, exercise physiologists, and dietary experts.
  - Assess the relationship between the various manifestations of metabolic syndrome and BPH/LUTS.
- Develop preventive strategies aimed at the underlying common pathophysiology of benign prostate disease.
- Develop studies that assess disease "phenotypes" and lead to better disease definitions (e.g., size versus morphological characteristics and their relative importance in producing symptoms, obstructive versus irritative symptoms relative to prostate morphology and size, and CP/CPPS patient phenotypes relative to urologic symptom profiles).

- Encourage the study of primary prevention for CP/CPPS and BPH/LUTS.
- Develop a plan for a multidisciplinary working group to develop a specific research agenda for symptom and health status measurement related to male LUTS.
  - Include investigators interested in the broad spectrum of underlying conditions, as well as the developers of the prominent instruments.
  - Invite professional societies, national and international, and other Government organizations to participate.
- Develop a collaborative network to standardize treatment assessment.
  - Create a LUTS Treatment Collaborative Network that would allow the critical aggregation of thought leaders, trial design experts, industrial collaborators, and various Federal agencies to identify clinically meaningful assessments of promising medical, minimally invasive, and surgical treatments.

www.ingramcontent.com/pod-product-compliance
Lightning Source LLC
Chambersburg PA
CBHW081551170526
45166CB00009B/2663